Psychiatric Nursing Revisited
The Care Provided for Acute Psychiatric Patients

Psychiatric Nursing Revisited
The Care Provided for Acute Psychiatric Patients

Ray Higgins, Keith Hurst and Gerald Wistow
Nuffield Institute for Health
University of Leeds

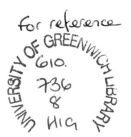
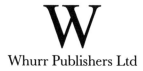

Whurr Publishers Ltd

© 1999 Whurr Publishers Ltd
First published 1999 by
Whurr Publishers Ltd
19b Compton Terrace, London N1 2UN, England

Reprinted 2000

British Library Cataloguing in Publication Data
A catalogue record for this book is available from the British
Library.

ISBN 1 86156 086 9

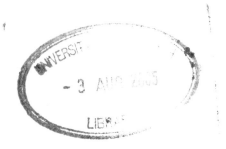

Printed and bound in the UK by Athenaeum Press Ltd,
Gateshead, Tyne & Wear

Contents

Acknowledgements   ix

Chapter 1   1
Psychiatric Nursing Revisited – An Overview

Chapter 2   13
Setting the Scene
Historical Overview
Recent Context
Slow Progress Towards Community Care
Rising Demand for Services
Overview of Nursing Practice
Summary

Chapter 3   29
Research Methods
Selection of Fieldwork Sites
Statistical Profile of Fieldwork Sites
Pre-pilot and Pilot Studies
Main Study
Non-participant Observation of Ward Staff and Patients
Analysing Fieldwork Data
Postal Survey
Feedback Seminars for Fieldwork Sites
Summary

Chapter 4   43
The Hospital Care Context
Ward Environments

Summary of the Features of Fieldwork Sites
Summary of the Ward Characteristics
Patient Populations
Features of Patient Populations
Discussion
Summary

Chapter 5   **67**

Management and Leadership
Staff Cover
Organisational Arrangements
Service Development
Staff Support
Stress and Staff Sickness
Clinical Supervision
Barriers to Effective Management and Leadership
Responsibility, Accountability and Authority
Paperwork and Administrative Duties
Summary

Chapter 6   **94**

Caring for Patients
Admission to Hospital
Risk Assessment and Management
Benefits of Hospitalisation
Admission Procedures
The Care Process
Therapeutic Relationship Between Named Nurse and Patient
Patients' Emotional Cues to which Nurses Respond
Nursing Care
Therapeutic Groupwork
Multidisciplinary Working
Communication and Counselling
Updating Care Plans
Other Ward Activities
The Role of Nursing Assistants
Basic and Continuing Education
The Nursing Contribution to Patient Care
Patients' Perceptions of Nursing Care
Discharge and Aftercare Arrangements
The Care Programme Approach
Summary

Chapter 7   147
Summary of Findings, Conclusions and Recommendations
Patient Populations
Basic and Continuing Education
Activities Performed by Ward Staff
Grade E and D Nurse Activity
Defensive Practice
Multidisciplinary Working
Grade A Nursing Assistants
Patients' Perceptions of Nursing Care
Implications for Policy and Practice

Appendix 1   159
National and Regional Statistics

Appendix 2   173
Trust Profile

Appendix 3   177
Ward Environment List

Appendix 4   180
Ward Manager Questionnaire

Appendix 5   184
Fieldwork Plan

Appendix 6   186
Manager and Nurse Interview Questions

Appendix 7   215
Glossary for Nurse and Patient Schedules

Appendix 8   224
Report on the Qualitative Pre-pilot Project

Appendix 9   232
Report on the Qualitative Pilot Project

Appendix 10   244
Patient Profile

Appendix 11   245
Nurse Activity and Personal Details Questionnaire

Appendix 12   253
Postal Survey of Trust Profiles

Appendix 13   260
Postal Survey of Ward Profiles and Operational Routines for Acute
Psychiatric Admission Wards

Appendix 14   274
Summary Reports from Feedback Seminars

Appendix 15   283
Additional Data for Text Figures

Bibliography   304

Index   315

Acknowledgements

Many individuals have been associated with the project over the past 3 years; their contributions and help have been invaluable. Among those who deserve special mention is Margaret Southwell, who did much to get the project on the road and who was involved in the early stages of the fieldwork. Our thanks are also extended to Angela Stewart, Tim Eager and Norma Doherty, who helped at the beginning of the study, and to Jenny Chin who undertook much of the data analysis.

We are immensely grateful to the members of our Research Advisory Group, who offered their support and constructive criticism throughout the research: Harry Cronin (Senior Nurse Manager [Mental Health], Wakefield and Pontefract Community NHS Trust), Jim Keown (Divisional Nurse Manager [Mental Health], City and Hackney Community NHS Trust), Simon Large (Executive Director of Planning, Leeds Community and Mental Health NHS Trust), Robert Macrowan (Nursing Officer, Department of Health), Maggie Pearson (formerly Professor of Health and Community Care, University of Liverpool and subsequently Director of R&D, North West Region), Jane Newson-Smith (Consultant Psychiatrist, St Mary's Hospital, Isle of Wight) and Liz Meerabeau (Nursing Liaison Officer, Department of Health) who chaired the Group. We are especially grateful to Dr Liz Scott of the Department of Health for commissioning the study. We also thank our colleagues at the Nuffield Institute, Brian Hardy and Mary Godfrey, who made extensive comments on a complete draft of the report. Margaret Henderson deserves special mention for her invaluable contribution to the main fieldwork.

We are particularly grateful to our funders, the Department of Health, and to all the staff at the 11 participating sites, without whose co-operation the study would not have been possible. The views expressed here are our own and not necessarily those of the Department of Health.

Chapter 1
Psychiatric nursing revisited – an overview

This chapter provides an overview of one detailed, empirical study of acute mental health nursing and patient activity research that joins a family of similar studies, for example Altschul (1972), Towell (1975), Cormack (1976, 1983), Faulkner *et al.* (1994) and Hurst (1993a, 1995a).

In Chapter 2, we explore why mental health has a high political profile in the 1990s, and how recent cases of mentally ill people committing violent offences have fuelled public anxiety about the dangers posed by a minority of mentally ill people. Since community care became the central plank of government policy for the care of mentally ill people, we explore its chequered history and why, because of community care's slow and uneven development, fresh impetus was given to the policy in the late 1980s.

Also in Chapter 2, we examine why community-based alternatives failed to keep pace with the decline in the number of psychiatric beds. By the early 1990s, this failure coincided with an apparent substantial rise in the demand for specialist mental health services. The pressure on remaining psychiatric beds became severe, and occupancy levels in excess of 100% became commonplace, especially in the larger urban areas and cities. Simultaneously, policy-makers and practitioners began to focus on the role of nursing in mental health services. This resulted in a review of mental health nursing and the publication in 1994 of *Working in Partnership: A Collaborative Approach to Care* (Department of Health, 1994a), the first review of such nursing since *Psychiatric Nursing: Today and Tomorrow* in 1968. We examine why both reports emphasise the importance of counselling and psychotherapeutic approaches to nursing care.

However, we note from the literature in Chapter 2 the relatively slow progress towards developing such approaches. Two principal obstacles are discussed:

- the dominance of the medical model in nursing, with its emphasis on monitoring patients' signs and symptoms;
- the changing patient mix in acute wards, which makes it difficult for nurses to practise counselling and other therapeutic approaches.

We explore why, despite the introduction of Project 2000 in 1989, nurse education problems continue, and why gaps in the provision of care compound mental health nurse education and practice problems. The nursing literature we review in Chapter 2 also identifies difficulties faced by nursing staff, including:

- the diversity of acute patients' needs;
- the infrequent contact between nurses and patients;
- the burden of paperwork on nurses, which partly relates to defensive practices that help to protect nurses from the consequences of untoward incidents.

In Chapter 3, we begin the search for evidence to explain the problems in modern mental health nursing. We analyse data from three former regional health authorities (RHAs) on the shift from hospital to community care for people with mental health problems. On the basis of this analysis, we show why the former RHAs of Yorkshire and Northern (Regions A and B) and sites in Inner London (Region C) were selected for fieldwork studies.

Next in Chapter 3, we explain how data from 11 sites in these regions were collected to examine the range of contexts in which nurses work. The data included those from:

- interviews conducted with 118 members of staff of all grades;
- interviews with 52 patients concerning their illnesses and how they spent their time in hospital;
- observations of ward staff and patients, both to validate what they reported at interview and also to give an indication of the range of activities in which patients and staff might be involved;
- postal surveys that provided a broad overview of the organisation, management and deployment of nurses and the nature of patient populations in acute psychiatric settings;
- two seminars held with managers and clinicians that: (a) provided participating sites with a summary of findings; (b) tested the validity of the research team's findings; and (c) helped the research team to formulate robust recommendations.

In Chapter 4, we use data from our extensive fieldwork to show variations in the:

- age, type and location of hospitals;
- shape and size of wards;
- types of accommodation available to patients.

Next, we turn to patient populations and analyse them by:

- region;
- hospital's geographical location;
- hospital type;
- bed occupancy;
- gender ratio;
- age;
- previous admissions;
- length of stay;
- ethnic composition;
- severity of illness.

These data are examined in detail to throw light on modern psychiatric nursing. In Chapter 4, we provide evidence that supports the widely held perceptions of those working in acute mental health services that they increasingly care for more difficult patients. We distinguish between sites with 'difficult' and with more 'manageable' patient populations. The influence of patients on the nature of the nursing work, one of the most significant effects, is analysed. We also consider changing patient populations and the impact on nurses' workloads in the light of:

- increased pressure on beds;
- beds increasingly being blocked;
- an increased severity of patients' illness in wards;
- more detained patients being in wards.

Next, we turn to why staff caring for difficult patients reported less job satisfaction. We show that stabilising patients' conditions prior to discharge, rather than nurses' involvement in the complete process of care, became the norm, and how one consequence of the change in patient populations – nurses' contact time with patients – was squeezed.

We explore a potential *bête noire* of nurses – the volume of paperwork and additional administrative duties regarded by nurses as a burden. The reasons behind these workload pressures, said to limit patients' involvement in care planning, are discussed. Two main nursing dilemmas are included in the chapter:

1. allowing patients sufficient time to recover before discharge, and discharging patients too early, thereby maintaining a steady turnover of patients to release beds;
2. the increasing tension between a custodial and a therapeutic approach to care.

We go on to examine more favourable aspects of psychiatric nursing that create job satisfaction. Staff caring for more manageable populations were generally able to maintain what they regarded as a more satisfying nursing role. This preferred role, a nursing process-based one, allowed them sufficient time with patients for care-planning and preparing them adequately for discharge to a therapeutic environment.

The other noticeable differences between regions in terms of difficult and manageable patient populations are described in Chapter 4. Thus Region C sites cared for demonstrably more difficult populations than did Region B sites. We noticed that, even though staffing arrangements had been adjusted to deal with more severely ill patients, the pressure on beds meant that staff were often unable adequately to undertake the complete process of care; their overriding concern was to free beds to make way for patients with more immediate needs. In contrast, Region B had one of the smallest reductions in bed numbers of any region and also one of the highest increases in hospital nursing staff numbers. As a result, staff were apparently more able to deal with the demands imposed on them and be involved in the complete process of care.

Next in Chapter 4, we turn to nurse education and explore why nurses – including staff only recently qualified – said that much of their basic education was largely divorced from the work that they carried out in wards. In particular, we identify the emphasis in nurse education towards the physical aspects of nursing, relatively little attention being paid to mental health issues. This perceived bias was linked to the dominance of the medical model, with its focus on checking the signs and symptoms of illness. The development of nursing models, with their emphasis on viewing patients holistically, counterbalances this dominance. Although bias had been partly addressed by the introduction of Project 2000-based curricula, the lack of practical experience in acute psychiatric wards during basic education meant that newly qualified nurses were often unprepared for what they faced in the wards. We conclude that, as a result of a lack of preparation, these nurses often require extra supervision during the early months of their first appointment, thereby increasing the pressures on existing staff.

We note in Chapter 4 that, despite G and F grade nurses providing in-service education on aspects of nursing practice and policy developments, the principal method of developing skills and knowledge among experienced staff was their independent reading of nursing literature. We underline a related phenomenon: securing time to attend relevant courses to develop their skills often proved difficult for qualified staff. Cost was an important issue because staff increasingly had to pay course fees.

In Chapter 5, we explore nursing management and leadership. We show that G and F grade nurses were responsible for the ward management and clinical leadership. This involved ensuring that the ward was appropriately staffed and nurses adequately supported. We note that the G grade nurses were responsible for addressing inpatient needs by carefully compiling duty rotas. We explore why this activity is considered unduly time-consuming because of the number of factors that duty rota compilers have to consider, for example internal rotation as the principal means of organising staff cover, and staff who belonged to a nursing team that related to a consultant psychiatrist.

Several encouraging aspects are discussed Chapter 5:

- Primary nursing operated in all sites.
- Named nurses were linked to individual patients' care plans, and patients were involved throughout.
- Named nurses were responsible for feeding back information concerning patients' progress to other members of the multidisciplinary care team at weekly meetings.

However, in Chapter 5, we go on to explore a number of difficulties with implementing and operating primary nursing.

Later in the chapter, we show from fieldwork how senior nurses are responsible for developing and implementing policies that address particular nursing issues and ensure that staff have the requisite skills to carry out policies. Owing to the demanding nature of patients in some sites and the volume of paperwork that nurses were required to complete, it was often difficult for senior nurses to adopt a proactive, planned approach to service and staff development. We were concerned, therefore, that the pressures on staff were taking a heavy toll and resulted in an unexpected increase in staff sickness. As a result, adjustments to staffing arrangements, including staff working their days off to cover for sick colleagues, were often required at short notice. We reveal that many nurses admitted taking sick leave because of ward pressures, although recourse to this coping strategy was taken with great reluctance. Senior nurses, monitoring staff sickness, reported a trend – a rise in the level of short-term staff sickness – when particularly difficult patients were admitted. Even more worrying, some also reported increasing staff turnover at these difficult times.

A system of individual performance review operated in all sites. Appraisal involved an examination, usually at monthly intervals, of the clinical work and developmental needs of individual staff. Unfortunately, owing to pressures on their time, many senior nurses had difficulty supervising and appraising staff.

Later in Chapter 5, we explore other barriers to effective management and leadership. We note that devolving responsibilities to ward level had a significant impact on senior ward nurses' roles, to the extent that their managerial and administrative duties increasingly conflicted with their role as senior clinicians. We also consider explanations for the striking decrease in the time that G and F grade nurses spent in direct (face-to-face) patient care and the remarkable increase in time spent in associated (mostly hotel/administrative) work.

Despite these alarming data, we show that devolution of managerial and administrative responsibilities has, although complex and uncertain, positive as well as negative effects on ward management and leadership. We note that the freedom senior nurses enjoy to develop ward services is welcomed. In contrast, however, the increase in administrative duties is vehemently disliked. Having the autonomy to exercise discretion was closely related to the pace and nature of devolution. In Region A especially, senior nurses often had the responsibility, but their ability to act autonomously was limited compared with Region C and, and to a lesser degree, Region B, where direct control over the ward budget helped ward managers to exercise responsibility, authority and independence.

Another phenomenon emerges in Chapter 5. Senior nurses' increased responsibilities have changed the nature of their professional relationships, particularly with medical staff. We show how the traditional pattern of medically led decision-making has shifted to one in which nursing inputs are increasingly important. The notion of shared accountability and the move to multidisciplinary working is a significant development. In Region C, in particular, where bed occupancy levels were high and pressure on beds severe, senior nurses challenged some medical decisions, especially those relating to ward admissions, on the grounds of safety for staff and patients in the ward.

Notwithstanding the dilemma that senior nurses encounter in relation to the balance between clinical and administrative roles, many in Regions B and C had obtained managerial qualifications, although few had received specific education or, in their view, adequate preparation for their management role. We test whether nurses view their large managerial workloads positively or whether their administrative duties are seen as a burden. We carefully analyse the data and conclude that senior nurses identify a strong link between their greater responsibilities for the ward and the increase in administrative duties. All G and F grade nurses reported that between 50% and 66% of the paperwork they completed was not directly relevant to patient care, was often routine and was completed for the benefit of others. Understandably, this is an aspect of their work with which nurses were least satisfied.

In Chapter 6, we shift the focus to patient care. Despite difficulties in modern, acute mental health nursing, we show that nurses have a deep regard for acute psychiatric patients. Nurses identify four principal reasons for admitting psychiatric patients to hospitals:

1. risk of harm to self or others;
2. self-neglect;
3. inability to cope with everyday activities;
4. non-compliance with prescribed medication.

In our study, a significant proportion of admissions were emergencies, many being associated with alcohol or drug abuse, particularly among young men. Such abuse is identified as a factor contributing to more difficult patient populations. Severe pressure on beds and a lack of suitable alternative facilities for treating severely ill people meant that the threshold for what was an acceptable risk for admission had been lowered. Nurses and patients said that the principal benefits of hospital care were:

• to stabilise an individual's condition;
• to provide a safe environment;
• to provide time out and refuge for those no longer able to cope;
• to address the underlying causes of patients' problems.

Professionals in our study felt that, ideally, a doctor and a nurse should jointly carry out the admission procedure to prevent patients repeating information and duplicating effort. In practice, however, we saw that it was usual for a nurse to begin the admission process alone.

After recording a new patient's personal details, the nurse conducted an initial assessment of the patient's mental state. Later, the doctor would also ask the patient for personal details, carry out a physical examination, make an initial diagnosis and, if necessary, prescribe medication. The admitting doctor and nurse might also independently obtain information from anyone accompanying the patient about the circumstances precipitating admission. If the patient had been admitted under a section of the 1983 Mental Health Act, the nurse checked that the paperwork was in order. We were not surprised to observe admission procedures taking more than 1 hour.

Allocation of a new patient to a named nurse was usually to the admitting nurse. However, we note in Chapter 6 that, if the patient had been in hospital before, he or she might be assigned to a particular nurse known to him or her. As named nurses, E and D grade staff were regarded as the linchpins of patient-centred care. The success of the nurse–patient relationship largely depends upon the psychotherapeutic and interpersonal skills of the nurse. Three elements comprise the therapeutic relationship, in which the skills of nurses are used:

* establishing trust between nurse and patient;
* encouraging patients' motivation;
* providing support to patients.

Information about patients, especially recent changes in a patient's behaviour, was obtained during shift hand-overs. From the fieldwork data analysed in Chapter 6, we note a number of emotional cues from patients that triggered responses from nurses. Consequently, contact between nurses and patients occurred infrequently and was generally *ad hoc* and of short duration. Nurses said that this was inevitable owing to the unpredictability of many interactions with patients in acute wards.

Nurses' intuition-based interpretation of verbal and non-verbal cues was also used when caring for patients. Expert interpretation was developed through the experience of contact with patients over a number of years. There were more structured nurse–patient interactions, most notably those associated with care planning. However, the inherently unpredictable nature of mental health nursing meant that nurse–patient discussions often had to be rescheduled. Rising pressures on nurses' time meant that they increasingly dealt with the most demanding or ill patients, others being left to their own devices.

The different nursing models of patient care used across the fieldwork sites, and the similarities in the approaches adopted, are explored in Chapter 6. We note how the nursing assessment was carried out at the time of admission or soon after. This entailed discussing with the patient his or her:

- mental state;
- social circumstances;
- physical well-being;
- spiritual state.

The care plan consisted of:

- a description of the patient's problems;
- activities in which the patient was involved;
- an analysis of the success of particular nursing interventions (based on discussions with the patient);
- reasons for any changes in the care plan.

We are encouraged to note in Chapter 6 how patients were motivated to be actively involved in the development of care plans. However, the initial assessment and care plan developed at or soon after admission was often produced by the nurse with little input from the patient because many patients were too ill to participate.

Next, we delve into the way in which care plans are used to address problems, plan an appropriate response and evaluate the success of particular nursing interventions. Some care involved the patient attending group activities organised by occupational therapists or ward staff. Care also involved discussing an individual patient's progress in the weekly multidisciplinary care team (MDT) meeting. Despite the emphasis on multidisciplinary working, however, little appeared to occur outside weekly meetings. Interprofessional working meant nothing more than the named nurse chasing colleagues to see whether they had acted on decisions taken at the MDT meeting, particularly in terms of the care programme approach (CPA).

Later in Chapter 6, we return to record-keeping. We explore the growth of paperwork handled by nursing staff and their decreasing hands-on involvement with patients. We also analyse nursing activity analysis data from a number of perspectives. From these data and analyses we:

- attempt to reconcile the dilemma between direct patient care and completing paperwork;

- consider the increased stress and sickness among staff in relation to these data;
- explore the limited access to secretarial or IT support for recording information;
- consider the lack of integrated or computerised patient notes containing the records of all professionals involved in patient care.

Next in Chapter 6, we turn to nursing assistants and the valuable support they give to qualified staff, especially as pressures on qualified nurses increase. We note that despite unqualified staff having fewer administrative tasks, thereby spending more of their time with patients, their direct care time, like that of their qualified nurse counterparts, is falling. Despite this, nursing assistants are acquiring a significant nursing care role:

- operating as associate workers to named nurses;
- undertaking close observational work of patients;
- performing aspects of admission procedures and care planning.

In Chapter 6, we discuss how most patients have the highest praise for nurses and nursing care. The value of support provided by named nurses and the opportunity for patients to talk to someone who did not judge their words or actions is an important encouraging finding. We consider patients' understanding of care planning and how no patient held or had a copy of his or her care plan, and few recalled having seen it. These issues did not, however, worry the patients. Patients accept nurses' writing about their progress as a necessary part of being in hospital.

We go on to explore in Chapter 6 how a lack of 'quality time' with nurses contributes to inpatients' boredom. Nurses' paperwork and the general pressure on staff were commonly said to limit nurse–patient interaction. Our analysis shows that staff spent little time with patients – 4% compared with the 28% that patients spent doing nothing, watching television or undertaking their own personal care.

Finally in Chapter 6, we discuss discharge and aftercare. We explore how:

- ideally, discharge consists of gradually increasing lengths of leave until discharge, and how, after each period of leave, the named nurse and patient discuss successes and failures;
- this information was fed back to colleagues at the next MDT meeting;

- for patients who were only in hospital a few days, discharge processes were less elaborate;
- nurses at a number of sites felt that, owing to pressures on beds, some patients were sent on leave or discharged too early and with insufficient preparation.

CPA is explored in Chapter 6. CPA operated in all sites, although in some it had only recently been fully implemented. We show that, despite few staff receiving specific education in this new approach, CPA was offered to most patients where discharge was considered. During fieldwork, we noted that CPA consisted of a checklist of actions and that it was the role of the named nurse to ensure that the checklist was completed. Consideration for inclusion on the supervision register was part of the discussion of the CPA before individuals left hospital and at care programme reviews following discharge. The aim of the register was, we saw, to identify those people at risk and ensure that local services focused on these patients. We also observed that few individuals were registered and noted that no patient interviewed knew that the register existed.

Owing to the CPA issues in Chapter 6, we compare the benefits of CPA arrangements with previous discharge procedures. Most important of all, we note, was that patients had an aftercare plan organised before leaving hospital. A major drawback of CPA, however, was the volume of paperwork it generated from nurses. CPA also meant that nurses spent a considerable time sharing information with other professionals, organising and attending meetings, and ensuring that all the elements of a patient's care programme were in place prior to discharge. We show that a number of sites had attempted to reduce the burden of extra administration and meetings by combining CPA discussions with weekly MDT meetings. The care co-ordination aspect of the CPA is a new role for nurses. Consequently, this involved much behind-the-scenes work liaising with others to ensure the successful implementation of the CPA for individual patients.

However, we tease out the reasons why professionals felt that the main problem with CPA was the lack of integration of hospital CPA procedures with social service department care management systems. This resulted in nurses undertaking aspects of discharge that they felt should be carried out by local authority care managers.

In Chapter 7, we draw the findings together and underline the principal messages and implications for those agencies responsible for mental health policy and practice:

- health authorities;
- social services;
- health and social services authorities jointly;
- service providers;
- nurse educators.

We show that, by extension, many of these messages have clear implications for those at the centre responsible for such services.

We also show how recommendations relating nurse education and workforce planning need to take account of the full cycle of mental illness. Thus solutions appropriate for an acute setting may not be achievable without changes in other settings. In order to ensure continuity of care and treatment, such recommendations also need to take account of skill mix and grade mix, expertise, overlap and support available in the community. We underline these recommendations by pointing out how users often speak of dislocation from other support systems when admitted to hospital.

We argue that, if appropriate skill and grade mixes are to be achieved, the skills required to care for individuals need to be considered separately from those required to treat patients. We see that nurses traditionally undertake both activities. However, we consider that caring – for example keeping patients occupied and comfortable in Maslow's terms – does not require scarce higher-level nursing skills. We contrast this view with the belief that the treatment of patients, such as by therapeutic counselling, does require the skills of experienced nurses. Our rationale is that the lack of separation of higher-level from lower-level nursing knowledge and skills contributes to the increased pressures on nurses as they work in increasingly stressful environments. If there is an accumulation of skills in such settings, we argue that the lack of transferability of skills is a reason why there is an overdemand for inpatient services. We argue in Chapter 7 that many patients have repeat inpatient episodes because of the lack of acute mental health skills in other settings, and small numbers of patients often account for very high inpatient usage.

Finally, we show our concern in Chapter 7 that if nurses are taught to cope with pressures, then there is an implicit acceptance of the pressure, and it is unlikely that either causes or solutions will be unearthed. In the light of these discussions, we return to patient flows, demand, case mix and strengthening of the hospital–community interface to show how nursing can be managed more effectively.

Chapter 2
Setting the scene

Mental health is currently high on the political agenda (Bottomley, 1994; Malone, 1995; Department of Health, 1996a; National Health Service Executive, 1996). The renewed impetus given to community care and mental health services emerges from the White Paper *Caring for People* and subsequent policy guidance (Department of Health, 1989, pp. 55–8; 1990a, pp. 75–83). Also, the Health of the Nation initiative (Department of Health, 1992a) identifies the reduction of mental illness mortality and morbidity as one of five key areas along-side coronary heart disease, strokes, cancers, accidents, and HIV/AIDS and sexual health (Department of Health, 1993).

Moreover, recent cases of violent offences committed by mentally ill people in particular, such as those concerning Christopher Clunis (Department of Health, 1994b), Andrew Robinson (Blom-Cooper *et al.*, 1995) and the Woodley Team inquiry (Woodley Team Report, 1995) into the homicide committed by a person suffering with a severe mental illness, have received much publicity and increased public anxiety about the potential danger posed by a minority of mentally ill people to the community (Audit Commission, 1994; House of Commons Health Committee, 1994; Mental Health Foundation, 1994; Mental Health Act Commission, 1995).

These concerns emerged despite data pointed out by a House of Commons Health Committee report (1994, p. xvi) that there is a far higher risk of a mentally ill person committing self-harm than harming others:

the risk of suicide is about 100 times greater than the risk of violence to others

and that the best predictor of violence is a history of such behaviour, whether or not they are mentally ill. Additionally, many reports paint a bleak picture of overburdened local services, raising doubts about staff's abilities to cope satisfactorily with current demand (Audit Commission, 1994; Department of Health, 1994a, 1996a; House of Commons Health Committee, 1994; Mental Health Foundation, 1994; Mental Health Act Commission, 1995; National Health Service Executive, 1996).

This chapter, therefore, briefly describes the literature about mental health nursing and provides an introduction to:

- the context in which nurses operate;
- the pressures experienced by staff working in acute psychiatric admission wards;
- what nursing care provided to patients actually consists of.

The main issues raised are examined in detail in the main body of the text. Similarities and differences between findings recorded in the present study, compared with those expressed in earlier nursing studies, are also discussed. First, an historical overview is given concerning the development of mental health policy since the 1950s.

Historical overview

Central government emphasis on community care as the pivotal policy for those with mental health problems is said to date from a speech given by the then Health Minister, Enoch Powell, in 1961. In this speech, he announced the run-down, and eventual closure, of the large, remote, Victorian 'Water Tower', institution-type psychiatric hospitals. Official thinking had, however, been moving in this direction during the 1950s (Ministry of Health, 1954, 1956). In 1962 *The Hospital Plan* was published, which confirmed the shift in post-war policy on mental health services from an institution-based policy to one that emphasised community care alternatives (Tooth and Brooke, 1961; Ministry of Health, 1962).

After the 1960s, a broad consensus developed that community care was a more appropriate and more cost-effective form of care for those with mental health problems (Department of Health and Social Security, 1968; Jones 1972; Butler 1993). The poor standards of care for many long-term patients in psychiatric hospitals became increasingly evident. This was confirmed by a number of well-publicised inquiries and research studies during the 1960s and 70s (Goffman, 1961; Robb, 1967; Department of Health and Social Security, 1969, 1972, 1973; Morris, 1969; Martin, 1984). Proponents argued that community care should replace institutional care as the central plank of policy and service development. Several reasons were put forward to support this view:

- It would reduce the disabling and stigmatising effects of prolonged institutionalisation (Goffman, 1961; Martin, 1984).
- The availability of drugs enabled the management of many mental illnesses outside hospital (Jones, 1972).
- Research highlighted the benefits of treating and supporting people in their own homes and other community-based settings (Knapp *et al.*, 1992).
- There was a growing awareness of patients' rights and an emphasis on choice for service users (Department of Health and Social Security, 1983; Department of Health, 1989).

Community care was supported on economic grounds and institutional care rejected as being expensive. According to the Audit Commission (1986, 1994), many people currently in psychiatric hospitals could be cared for at less than half the cost in a non-institutional alternative setting.

The economic argument was a principal driving force behind community care policies developed in the 1980s. However, the reduced cost argument is not as clear cut. Providing care for the proportion of people with severe and enduring mental illnesses who require considerable support and care can be costly in community settings (Netten and Beecham, 1993). Nevertheless, resettlement of the long-stay hospital population was encouraged because *Caring for People* suggested that, as psychiatric hospitals were closed, the proceeds from the sale of buildings and land should be used to develop community facilities (Department of Health, 1989, paras 7.10–7.12). This view was reiterated by the Chief Executive of the NHSE, Alan Langlands (Higgins and Wistow, 1994).

The 1975 White Paper *Better Services for the Mentally Ill* (Department of Health and Social Security, 1975) distinguished between long-stay beds for patients with enduring mental illness and acute, short-stay beds for patients having serious but short-lived crises. The former were to be supported in their own homes and other community residential settings, additional support being provided by local health and social care services (Griffiths, 1988; Department of Health, 1989, 1990a). However, the White Paper recognised that short-term specialist hospital services would still be required for those experiencing acute illness crises. These services were to be located in the psychiatric units of district general hospitals (Department of Health and Social Security, 1975).

Recent context

The aim of recent mental health policy has been to target specialist psychiatric services on the most severely ill people to ensure that they receive treatment, care and follow-up, and to maintain their contact with health and social services. A CPA for the assessment, co-ordination and review of care for individuals, and a specific grant to local authorities to address the social care needs of people with serious mental illness – the Mental Illness Specific Grant (MISG), £31m in 1992/93 – were introduced in 1991 to provide further support for people in the community (Department of Health, 1989, 1990b). CPA was supplemented by supervision registers introduced in 1994 for those most at risk of violence to others or themselves, or at risk of self-neglect, or who needed particular care and follow-up after leaving hospital.

Slow progress towards community care

At one level, emphasis on community-based solutions to caring for the mentally ill has been a great success, resulting in a steady decline in the number of psychiatric beds since the 1950s. Forty years on, the number of beds dropped by approximately two-thirds, from 149 000 in 1955 to 50 278 in 1991/92 (Audit Commission, 1994, p. 6; Davidge et al., 1993, 1994).

The resettlement of old long-stay residents from traditional asylums presented relatively few problems where this was part of a planned programme of reprovision and money had been transferred with individuals. People with challenging behaviour or severe physical impairments were more difficult to resettle and were often the last to be transferred to community settings. Consequently, a Mental Health Task Force was appointed in 1992 to add fresh momentum to the closure programme and to facilitate the development of a better range of quality community services because progress had slowed markedly during the 1980s (Audit Commission, 1986; Bottomley, 1994; Malone, 1995; Department of Health, 1996a). According to a recent Audit Commission (1994) report, part of the explanation for the slow progress was that approximately 66% of the expenditure on adult mental health services remained tied to the hospital sector: a total expenditure of £1.8 billion in 1992/93 (p. 7). Only £185 million (10%) was spent by local authorities, including a specific grant of £31 million. The remaining 24% was spent by the NHS on day hospital and community services.

Rising demand for services

A more worrying development arose during the 1980s. As the number of psychiatric beds continued to fall, there was a substantial rise in the demand for specialist mental health services. Owing to the slow development of replacement community services, acute psychiatric wards took the full brunt of meeting the demand.

The House of Commons Health Committee Report *Better off in the Community? The Care of People who are Seriously Mentally Ill* (House of Commons Health Committee, 1994, p. xii) noted that 'there is demonstrable pressure on acute beds in some areas'. A number of possible reasons for such pressures were given:

- a lack of suitable accommodation;
- the closure of long-stay psychiatric hospitals;
- the closure of district beds;
- the increased psychiatric morbidity in cities;
- inefficient bed management practices;
- inadequate community support staff;
- the ineffectiveness of joint health and social services discharge arrangements.

Whatever the cause, high bed occupancy rates in acute wards were noted by professional organisations, including the Royal College of Psychiatrists. In 1990 the average bed occupancy in Greater London psychiatric admission units was 95.7%, and over 100% in a third of units. The College's recommended average occupancy, on the other hand, was 85% (House of Commons Health Committee, 1994; Powell *et al.*, 1995). The Mental Health Act Commission (1995) raised concerns about the number of patients admitted compulsorily under the 1983 Mental Health Act. More than 40% of admissions in urban areas were detained patients, and in some wards this figure was 80% or more. Additionally, private beds and out-of-district beds became the means of alleviating the pressure in acute wards (Audit Commission, 1994; House of Commons Health Committee, 1994; Mental Health Foundation, 1994; Mental Health Act Commission, 1995).

One result of these pressures was a reduction in the overall length of patient stay, and inpatients being sent home on extended leave (Audit Commission, 1994). Consequently, the 1995 Mental Health (Patients in the Community) Act (Department of Health, 1995a) addressed the issue of extended leave by the introduction of supervised discharge as part of CPA arrangements. Another consequence of the explosion in demand was that many so-called new long-term patients – who had in the past languished in the wards of psychiatric hospitals – were inappropriately placed in acute wards, where other more needy patients could be treated. These developments compounded pressure on beds in some areas as a proportion of beds became blocked (Audit Commission, 1994; House of Commons Health Committee, 1994; Mental Health Act Commission, 1995).

The changing context of acute care is examined in this book, and its key features, with respect to 11 sites in three regions, are discussed. Against this background of greater pressures on staff working in acute units, the nature of nursing care is also examined (Chapters 5 and 6). However, a brief overview of the changing context and the nature of nursing care, noted in the nursing literature, is now provided.

Overview of nursing practice

Community care has remained the central plank of successive governments' policy towards those with mental health problems. Policymakers and practitioners have recognised that there remains a need for short-term crisis inpatient care for those unable or unwilling to cope in the community. The role and nature of mental health nursing, including hospital care, has been the subject of two major reviews since the 1960s namely:

*   *Psychiatric Nursing: Today and Tomorrow* (Ministry of Health, 1968);
*   *Working in Partnership: A Collaborative Approach to Care* (Department of Health, 1994a).

Mental health nursing education and skills

Both reports focused on the skills and training required by nurses in caring for patients. *Psychiatric Nursing: Today and Tomorrow* emphasised the importance of counselling and psychotherapeutic skills, and the education of individuals concerning the signs and symptoms of impending crises, in the belief that such an approach might reduce the likelihood of hospital admission. The authors of *Working in Partnership* – the Mental Health Nursing Review Team – reaffirmed the emphasis on counselling but also recognised the impact on nursing of the context in which wards were located.

A subgroup of the Standing Nursing and the Standing Mental Health Advisory Committees carried out a review of mental health nursing and produced the report *Psychiatric Nursing: Today and Tomorrow* (Ministry of Health, 1968). The Committee was asked to describe present practice and to prescribe the future development of mental health nursing. It was given the following terms of reference:

> To consider the functions of psychiatric nursing staff and having regard to the changing pattern of psychiatric treatment to make recommendations, in the first instance on nursing staff patterns in wards and departments of hospitals for the mentally ill and psychiatric units in general hospitals. (para. 1)

Best practice in mental health nursing was described as 'listening to and counselling patients' (para. 166). This reflected the greater emphasis placed on the nurses' role in supporting and counselling patients through current difficulties in preparation for their return to community living.

Thus the future of mental health nursing was to develop such practice, because:

> nursing staff will be required to play a more active, therapeutic role and ... they should be prepared accordingly ... Some existing forms of treatment, for example, behaviour therapy and aversion therapy, which are at present employed on a small scale may develop further and be employed more widely ... We think selected nurses will be trained to give psychological treatments to both individual patients and groups of patients. (para. 186)

Furthermore:

> some psychiatric nurses in this country will also develop advanced clinical roles, probably in a research setting and will signpost lines of development for psychiatric nursing in this country. (para. 187)

and:

> Acute mental illness units will demand more psychological skills and in particular, group psychotherapy. (para. 192)

The report recommended that basic and continuing education for nurses should reflect the greater need for counselling and psychotherapeutic approaches to patient care that would be required in the future:

> There should be experimental courses at basic and higher levels with a view to preparing nurses for an advanced clinical role. (para. 202)

Changes to nurse training should run in parallel with a research programme, which examines the 'psychotherapeutic role of the nurse' (para. 223).

In reaching their conclusions, the committee relied heavily on published work, such as that of Goddard and Goddard (1955), Oppenheim and Eeman (1955) and especially John (1961). John's emphasis on 'therapeutic nursing care' (p. 100) had a particularly significant influence on those responsible for producing *Psychiatric Nursing: Today and Tomorrow*. John described the treatments offered to psychiatric patients as either physical or psychotherapeutic:

> Physical treatment comprised such techniques as electro-convulsive therapy (ECT), deep or modified insulin and the use of drugs. Psychotherapy – seriously restricted by the shortage of medical and nursing staff – most frequently took the form of individual interviews, whilst attempts at group therapy were occasionally witnessed. (p. 37)

John identified a number of trends suggesting that the role and function of the mental health nurse needed to change because of advances in the armoury of drugs at the disposal of nurses and medical staff to treat mental illness. Such developments had transformed the skills needed by mental health nurses:

> Tranquillisers have certainly made patients more accessible to psychotherapy; they have controlled, to a large extent, aggressive and bizarre behaviour and, as a result, they have placed on the nurse's shoulders an ever increasing responsibility to persevere in attempts to achieve a therapeutic relationship. (p. 41)

Despite John's evidence, endorsed in *Psychiatric Nursing: Today and Tomorrow* that nurses needed to develop a counselling and psychotherapeutic role, later studies continued to report that such a role was practised to only a limited extent by nurses because the required realignment in nurse training was slow to be implemented (Altschul, 1972; Briggs, 1972; Towell, 1975; Cormack, 1976, 1983; Nolan, 1990, 1991a, 1991b, 1991c, 1993; Department of Health, 1994a). The principal reasons cited in studies to account for the slow progress in developing such an approach were the following:

- Nurse training was rooted in a medical model, which concentrated on signs and symptoms, leaving nurses ill-equipped to act as counsellors or psychotherapists (Altschul, 1972; Towell, 1975; Cormack, 1983; MacIlwaine, 1983; Carpenter, 1989; Nolan, 1990, 1991a, 1991b, 1991c, 1993).
- The medical model, with its narrow focus on current symptoms,

determined the short-term nature of many nurse–patient interactions (Altschul, 1972; Towell, 1975; Cormack, 1976, 1983). Moreover, Carpenter (1989) argued that nurses merely 'acted as agents of medical staff' (p. 22), for example dispensing medication and reporting changes in patients' mood and behaviour.

- Interactions between nurses and patients were infrequent and *ad hoc*, with no clear picture of the emotional cues to which nurses responded (MacIlwaine, 1983). Forming personal relationships with patients was found to be a limited feature of a nurse's role (Altschul, 1972; Towell, 1975).
- Nurses were often concerned with maintaining patient conformity to the busy schedule of ward activities and, more generally, with keeping social order in the ward (Carpenter, 1989).

By the late 1980s, it became clear that pressures on ward staff, as a result of rising demand for specialist services, began to make therapeutic practices largely untenable in many acute wards operating at 100% or more bed occupancy (Audit Commission, 1994; House of Commons Health Committee, 1994; Mental Health Foundation, 1994; Mental Health Task Force, 1994; Mental Health Act Commission, 1995; Powell *et al.*, 1995).

Against the background of mounting evidence highlighting the slow and uneven progress towards developing the advanced clinical role envisaged by *Psychiatric Nursing: Today and Tomorrow*, and the changing context in acute settings described above, a review of mental health nursing was undertaken 25 years later. The Mental Health Nursing Review Team, led by Professor Butterworth, began its work in April 1992 and presented its report – *Working in Partnership: A Collaborative Approach to Care* – to the Secretary of State for Health in February 1994 (Department of Health, 1994a).

The terms of reference for the Review Team were:

> To identify the future requirements for skilled nursing care in the light of developments in the provision of services for people with mental illness. (p. vi)

In addition, the Team was to examine:

> the impact of changes in society and social policy since the late sixties, and their implications for practice, education, research and management in mental health nursing. (p. 4)

The Review Team said that if there was one recommendation arising from the report, it would be:

> Mental health nursing should re-examine every aspect of its policy and practice in the light of the needs of people who use services. (p. 5)

The Mental Health Nursing Review Team's report emphasised the nurse's focus on addressing the individual needs of patients and that patients should, wherever possible, be involved in the development of care plans. In short, care should be patient-centred and needs-led. Moreover, a collaborative approach to care by a multidisciplinary team, including nurses, should be the norm.

Working in Partnership reaffirmed the core skills of the mental health nurse as counselling, caring, rehabilitation and medication management (p. 17) and stated that:

> Nursing responses and interventions should be founded upon a sound understanding of the individuals in their care. (p. 18)

The Review Team acknowledged that the introduction of Project 2000 (UKCC, 1986, 1987) addressed many of the criticisms levelled at nurse education in *Psychiatric Nursing: Today and Tomorrow* and subsequent studies. However, concerns about mental health nurse education remained. The limited availability of specific courses for mental health nurses at post-registration level and the recruitment to mental health nursing were of special concern (Department of Health, 1994a, Recommendation 36). Also, nurses needed to be prepared for work in a spectrum of care settings, and the woeful inadequacy of the required diversity of care settings in many areas was recognised (Department of Health, 1996a; National Health Service Executive, 1996).

Management and leadership

The responsibility for the management and clinical leadership of nursing staff falls on G and F grade nurses. This involves ensuring that the ward is appropriately staffed and the nurses adequately supported. Previous studies showed that the management of ward services is in a state of flux, reflecting the more general condition of nursing services (Mangan, 1993; Palmer, 1993; Roberts, 1993; Stewart, 1993). The introduction of Griffiths-style general management and the move to flatter management structures from the mid-1980s (Griffiths, 1983) are identified as paving the way for responsibilities and decision-making to be devolved to ward managers.

A number of studies (Jones, 1990; Audit Commission, 1991; Roberts, 1993) suggested that the drive to reduce public sector organisations' overheads, particularly management and other administrative costs, had an impact on the NHS (Department of Health, 1996b). Senior ward nurses reported that resource centres, consisting of individual wards or groups of wards, had been created within their hospitals. Resource centres were to be responsible for all operational aspects, including many of the personnel and finance functions previously handled centrally.

Thus devolution of responsibilities to ward level had a significant impact on the role of senior ward nurses, to the extent that their managerial and administrative duties, particularly service development and clinical supervision, increasingly conflicted with their role as senior clinicians. It was questioned whether the de-layering of management structures within the health service had gone too far.

The pressure to adopt a primarily administrative rather than clinical role was overwhelming. The question of whether ward managers needed to be nurses had been raised in the literature (Audit Commission, 1991). Senior staff were concerned that their managerial and administrative duties might eventually squeeze the time for their role as clinical leaders and their involvement in hands-on patient care.

Caring for patients

This section examines the work of E and D grade staff in their role as named nurses for particular patients. In performing the named nurse role, the following activities are involved:

- admitting patients;
- undertaking the complete process of care: assessment, planning, implementation, and reviewing the care plan;
- attending to the discharge and aftercare arrangements for patients.

An overview of the principal issues mentioned in the literature about these aspects of caring for patients is provided below and examined later.

Admission to hospital

The most frequent explanation of why someone should be admitted was risk of harm to self or to others (Flannigan et al., 1994; Mental Health Act Commission, 1995).

A feature of many admissions is their emergency nature: ward staff have little advance warning before the arrival of a new patient. The Mental Health Act Commission (1995) raised concerns about the prevalent use of detention for such admissions and the fact that many of these admissions were linked with drug or alcohol abuse in men aged between 18 and 25 years, which often led to violence and management problems in the wards (Gournay, 1994; Powell *et al.*, 1995). The result is that ward staff are increasingly required to deal with difficult and unpredictable situations in their wards. This means that it is often hard for them to maintain a safe, let alone therapeutic, environment for patients in their care.

In this respect, the issue of what constitutes acceptable risk has been voiced (Dickson, 1995; Grounds, 1995; Lipsedge, 1995; Mental Health Act Commission, 1995; Moss, 1995; Vincent and Moss 1995; Vinestock, 1996). In an attempt to avert untoward incidents in the wards, a number of studies reported the development of pre-admission units in some hospitals. Here, medical and nursing staff attempt to ascertain whether patients admitted as an emergency are suited to open wards, or whether a more secure environment is appropriate (Dickson, 1995; Grounds, 1995; Vinestock, 1996).

The care process

Individualised care is identified as a linchpin of modern nursing (Department of Health, 1994a). It consists of four related activities (Peplau, 1952; Roy, 1984; Roper *et al.*, 1980):

1. Assessment entails gathering information about the patient and the circumstances surrounding his or her admission. It involves an examination of the patient's mental state, social circumstances, physical well-being and spiritual needs. These form the basis of the care plan, the second key element of nursing care.
2. The care plan is used to explore aspects of the patient's life in more detail in order to identify goals and related interventions. However, care plans have been widely debated with respect to their purpose, the frequency of their use and the quality of recorded information (McMahon, 1988; MacVicar and Swan, 1992; Department of Health, 1994b; Blom-Cooper *et al.*, 1995; Woodley Team Report, 1995). Patients are encouraged to take an active involvement in the development of their care plans, but patients' actual involvement is variable (McIver, 1991; Biehal, 1993; North *et al.*, 1993; Rogers *et al.*, 1993; Department of Health, 1994a).

3. Implementation of interventions negotiated between nurse and patient, with the objective of addressing identified need, is the third aspect of individualised care (Peplau, 1952; Roy, 1984; Roper *et al.*, 1980).
4. The final aspect of nursing care is evaluation of the success, or otherwise, of each intervention.

Multidisciplinary working and a consensus approach to patient care are reported to be widely practised (Skelton, 1994; Geoghegan, 1995; Snowdon, 1995; Watson, 1995). However, some commentators have questioned the extent to which multidisciplinary working operates outside the weekly MDT meeting or ward round (Hurst, 1995b). A number of studies report the difficulty that nurses have in isolating their contribution to patient care from that arising from other factors, such as:

• the effects of medication;
• the work of other members of the multidisciplinary care team;
• the fact that patients are away from the situations that precipitated their illness.

The difficulty of measuring nursing outcomes is also noted (Bond and Thomas, 1991; Thomas *et al.*, 1996).

The issue of whether discussions between nurse and patient concerning the care plan constitute counselling has also been debated in the literature. On the one hand, some commentators argue that, owing to a patient's short stay in hospital, it is inappropriate for nurses to delve too deeply into underlying causes of a patient's illness: that is seen as the role of others (Clarke *et al.*, 1991). On the other hand, different commentators suggest that counselling in relation to the patients' wants and needs is a central aspect of the nursing role (Smith, 1988; Department of Health, 1994a). As already mentioned, the increasingly difficult ward context often militates against its use, with crisis intervention being the predominant approach (Audit Commission, 1994; House of Commons Health Committee, 1994; Mental Health Foundation, 1994).

From the patient's perspective, a successful admission is partly related to the effectiveness of the nurse–patient relationship (Jack, 1995; Savage, 1995; Wright, 1995). Much depends on the skills employed by nurses. Among the most important include (Burnard, 1987a, 1987b; Engledow, 1987; Department of Health, 1994a; Gijbels and Burnard, 1995):

- the ability to display empathy;
- to be a good listener and communicator;
- to provide emotional support;
- to be available to value the patient's uniqueness.

The use of such skills is vital to develop a trusting relationship (Engledow, 1987) in which therapeutic conversations can occur between nurse and patient (Burnard, 1987b). Trusting relationships and therapeutic conversations ensure that the patient is supported and encouraged to overcome his or her current problems (Altschul, 1972; Burnard, 1985, 1987b; Howard, 1992; Gijbels and Burnard, 1995).

A frequent observation noted in the nursing literature about nurse–patient interactions is the difficulty nurses appear to have in specifying exactly what are the emotional cues of patients to which they respond. Such interactions are infrequent, short in duration and *ad hoc* (Altschul, 1972; Towell, 1975; Cormack, 1976, 1983; MacIlwaine, 1983; Smith, 1988; Howard, 1992). One explanation put forward for this situation is the changing context of acute wards in which nurses are now called upon to operate. The issue of nurses using their intuition to identify when a patient needs support has also been discussed in the literature (Benner, 1984; Hurst *et al.*, 1991; Hurst, 1993b).

While generally positive about their relationship with nurses, patients also mentioned the lack of time devoted to them (Audit Commission, 1991, 1994; House of Commons Health Committee, 1994; Mental Health Foundation, 1994). They said that nurses, as well as dealing with increasingly demanding patients in the ward, also spent a lot of time completing paperwork. This lack of contact with nurses results in patients' sense of boredom in hospital. Detained patients were often less enthusiastic about their relationship with nurses (Barnes *et al.*, 1990; Coid, 1993). The high incidence of appeals against detention is cited as evidence to support this position (Mental Health Act Commission, 1995).

Nursing assistants provide valuable support to the work of qualified staff. With few administrative duties to undertake, they spend most of their time with patients (Roberts, 1994; Workman, 1996). Concern has been expressed that, as pressures on nurses increase, unqualified staff may be carrying out tasks that they are neither adequately prepared for nor competent to undertake, for example acting as associate work-ers to a qualified named nurse and undertaking close observations of patients considered to be a risk to themselves or to others (Audit Commission, 1991, 1994; Royal College of Nursing, 1992; Roberts,

1994; Workman, 1996). However, the incidence of nursing assistants acquiring additional skills via NVQs is mentioned in the literature (Roberts, 1994).

Discharge and aftercare arrangements

The decision to discharge someone from hospital is taken by members of the multidisciplinary care team. However, it is the consultant psychiatrist who has the final say concerning whether or not an individual should be discharged. If discharge is considered appropriate, CPA comes into operation. A number of studies report that in some parts of the country, such as inner London and other inner-city areas, some patients may, owing to pressure on beds, be discharged too early or put on extended leave to make way for other needy users (Audit Commission, 1994; Hollander and Slater, 1994; House of Commons Health Committee, 1994; Powell *et al.*, 1995).

CPA was introduced in April 1991 (Department of Health, 1990b) to provide a framework for health and social care agencies to work together to establish the care and treatment of people in the community. The slow progress of the full implementation of CPA is noted (North *et al.*, 1993; Mental Health Foundation, 1994; Clinical Standards Advisory Group, 1995a, 1995b; Malone, 1995; Social Services Inspectorate, 1995). Moreover, a number of studies indicate that CPA is often applied conditionally to individuals who have been detained or who are considered to be at particular risk, rather than to everyone leaving hospital (North *et al.*, 1993; Schneider, 1993; Social Services Inspectorate, 1995).

As part of the CPA discussions, attention is given to whether individuals who are considered a risk to themselves or to others should be included in the local supervision registers introduced in April 1994 (Department of Health, 1994c). To date, few individuals appear to have been registered (Bottomley, 1994; Caldicott, 1994a, 1994b; Department of Health, 1994a, 1995b; Clinical Standards Advisory Group, 1995a, 1995b; Mental Health Act Commission, 1995).

The principal benefit associated with CPA is a more systematic and co-ordinated approach to discharge (North *et al.*, 1993; Social Services Inspectorate, 1995). Two principal drawbacks to CPA have, however, been identified. First is the lack of integration of the CPA arrangements (the lead responsibility lying with the health service) and the care management systems (the principal responsibility of the local authority). The resulting confusion means that hospital staff appear to carry out elements of care management and local authority staff aspects of CPA, thereby putting undue pressure on staff in the respective organisations (North *et al.*, 1993; Audit Commission, 1994; House of Commons Health Committee, 1994; Mental Health Foundation, 1994; Department of Health, 1995b; Social Services Inspectorate, 1995). Second, the administrative burden imposed on nurses and doctors because of the paper-heavy nature of CPA in many localities is noted (North *et al.*, 1993; Schneider, 1993; Department of Health, 1995b; Social Services Inspectorate, 1995). The paucity of education concerning the operation of CPA is also reported (North *et al.*, 1993; Schneider, 1993; Social Services Inspectorate, 1995).

Summary

- Mental health currently enjoys a high profile as a result of policy initiatives and public anxiety about violent offences committed by mentally ill people.
- Community care is the main policy in mental health. However, the combination of the slow build-up of community alternatives to hospital care, the decline in the number of beds in asylums and the rising demand during the 1980s increases pressures on the remaining specialist services, especially those offered by acute wards.
- In the light of the changing context of acute care, concerns continue to be voiced about the adequacy of basic and continuing nurse education.
- A number of issues are raised with respect to the process of care, including: the impact of emergency admissions; the lack of contact between nurses and patients owing to ward pressures; the way in which unqualified staff are shouldering greater responsibility for patient care; the relative absence of multidisciplinary working; and problems associated with the operation of CPA.

Chapter 3
Research methods

Evidence from mental health nursing literature and specialists' knowledge of mental health services demonstrated a widely held perception that patients were presenting with more severe illnesses and consequently that pressure on beds had increased. Ward pressures were perceived to have had a significant impact on nursing care, with more emphasis on crisis intervention and the stabilisation of patients than on nurses involving themselves in the complete process of care. Consequently, the Department of Health commissioned a detailed study of mental health, the aims of which were to investigate four issues:

1. the patient population in acute psychiatric settings and the extent of change in recent years;
2. the number, grade and qualifications of nursing staff in acute psychiatric wards;
3. the activities performed by nurses caring for patients;
4. patients' perceptions of their nursing care.

This chapter describes the research design and the methods used in the study. The approach is based on that developed and applied in previous nursing studies undertaken by the Nuffield Institute for Health (Hurst and Quinn, 1992; Southwell et al., 1993; Hurst, 1995a). The research design consisted of seven elements:

1. the selection of fieldwork sites;
2. a statistical profile of the fieldwork sites;
3. face-to-face interviews with nurses and patients;
4. non-participant observation of nurses and patients;
5. analysing fieldwork data;
6. postal survey;
7. feedback seminars for fieldwork sites.

Selection of fieldwork sites

An analysis of RHA data was undertaken to help to select the fieldwork sites. The purpose of this analysis was to identify variations
between RHAs and the shifts away from hospital to community care
for people with mental health problems. The following data were
analysed:

- number of psychiatric hospital beds;
- number of hospital and community mental health nurses;
- number of places in local authority and independent sector homes.

A summary of the analyses is provided below (see Appendix 1 for
details).

Number of psychiatric hospital beds

*Bed reduction/increase between 1988/89 and 1991/92 (Department of Health,
1992b)*

- Yorkshire recorded the largest reduction in the number of acute
  beds of any Region (–26% compared with the national average of
  –6%).
- SW Thames registered a slight increase in acute bed numbers (2%
  over the national average).
- Yorkshire, NE Thames and SE Thames recorded among the highest reductions in the number of long-stay beds (–39%, –49% and
  –48% respectively compared with the national average of –35%).
- Northern and NW Thames experienced among the lowest reductions in long-stay bed numbers (–23% and –16% respectively
  compared with the national average).

Beds per 100 000 population in 1991/92 (Department of Health, 1992b)

- Northern and SW Thames recorded among the highest numbers
  of acute and long-stay beds (acute beds 37 per 100 000 population
  and 41 per 100 000, and long-stay beds 37 per 100 000 and 59 per
  100 000 respectively, compared with the national averages of 29
  per 100 000 and 27 per 100 000 respectively).
- Yorkshire and SE Thames registered among the lowest rates of
  available acute and long-stay beds (acute beds 30 per 100 000 and
  28 per 100 000, and long-stay beds 20 per 100 000 and 17 per
  100 000 respectively compared with the national average).

- Yorkshire and SW Thames recorded among the largest number of closures (4 and 4 respectively compared with the national average of 2.7).
- Northern region did not close any hospital during the period.

Number of hospital and community mental health nurses

In terms of hospital mental health nursing staff reduction/increases between 1985 and 1988 (Department of Health, 1990c):

- SE Thames experienced the greatest reduction of any region (–32.3% compared with the national average of –0.3%);
- Northern registered among the highest increase (6.5% over the national average);
- Yorkshire experienced a reduction close to the national average (–0.4%).

With respect to community mental health nursing staff reduction/increase in numbers between 1987 and 1988 (Department of Health, 1990c):

- Yorkshire, NE Thames, NW Thames and SE Thames recorded some of the highest increases (10.8%, 19.5%, 12.3% and 17.1% respectively compared with the national average of 11.2%);
- Northern and SW Thames registered among the lowest increases (5.4% and 6.5% respectively compared with the national average).

Number of mental health places provided in local authority and independent sector homes

Data on the number of mental health places provided in all sectors per 100 000 population in 1990 (Department of Health, 1991) yielded the following:

- Yorkshire and Inner and Outer London recorded among the highest rates (35.0 per 100 000, 50.4 per 100 000 and 37.5 per 100 000 respectively compared with the national average of 30.7 per 100 000);
- Northern recorded one of the lowest rates (26.4 per 100 000 compared with the national average).

On the basis of these data, it was agreed that the study should be undertaken in the former RHAs of Yorkshire and Northern, and at sites in Inner London (referred to as Regions A, B and C respectively throughout the report). Yorkshire and Northern were chosen because they appeared to represent different ends of the spectrum of change within mental health services. That is, Yorkshire appeared to be well advanced in the shift away from hospital to community-based care, whereas Northern appeared to be one of the least advanced regions, but it had increased its hospital staffing.

The former Yorkshire RHA recorded one of the largest reductions in long-stay and acute bed numbers between 1988/89 and 1991/92; one of the largest number of Water Tower hospitals with 100 or more beds closed between 1961 and 1992; one of the highest increases in the number of community nursing staff but one of the lowest increases in number of hospital nursing staff between 1987 and 1988; and one of the highest rates of mental health places per 100 000 head of population provided in local authority and independent sector homes in 1990.

In contrast, the former Northern RHA recorded one of the lowest reductions in long-stay and acute bed numbers; did not close any Water Tower hospitals with 100 or more beds during the same period; had one of the lowest increases in community nursing staff but recorded one of the highest increases in number of hospital nursing staff; and had one of the lowest rates for mental health places in local authority and independent sector homes.

Inner London sites were included in the study at the request of the Department of Health because it was widely perceived that the capital's acute mental health services were under considerable pressure compared with those of other parts of the country.

Following the identification of regions representing different ends of this change spectrum, it was important to select fieldwork sites that reflected the range of contexts in which nursing staff worked, thereby revealing differences in patient populations and related working styles. The selection criteria were as follows (see Tables 4.3A–D and 4.4A–D for details):

* geographical location: urban and rural settings;
* hospital type: district general hospitals, traditional Water Tower psychiatric hospitals, private hospitals and other service situations;
* average bed occupancy: 100% or more and below 100%.

Consequently, in the light of the three criteria above, four fieldwork sites were selected in each region. One of the selected sites was unable, at a late stage, to proceed with the study, and it was not possible for it to be replaced in time. The 11 fieldwork sites are referred to as A1–4,

B5–8 and C9–11 throughout the report. The key characteristics of each site are discussed in Chapter 4, but in summary:

1. Geographical location:
   - urban sites (six): A1, A4, B7, C9, C10 and C11;
   - rural sites (five): A2, A3, B5, B6 and B8.
2. Hospital type:
   - four district general hospitals: A2, B7, B8 and C9;
   - three traditional Water Tower hospitals: A3, B6 and C11;
   - four other service settings, for example community units and stand-alone mental health units: A1, A4, B5 and C10.
3. Average bed occupancy level:
   - five with a bed occupancy level of 100% or above: A1, B5, C9, C10 and C11;
   - six with bed occupancies below 100%: A2, A3, A4, B6, B7 and B8.

The Chief Executive's permission was sought to carry out the study in each fieldwork site. Once permission had been granted by the Chief Executive, the approval of the Local Research Ethics Committee was sought. In the meantime, information about the study was sent to the mental health manager responsible for acute psychiatric services, and a preliminary discussion was held to identify a suitable ward to be involved in the study. It was left to the mental health manager to secure the agreement of the ward manager and staff to participate.

After Local Research Ethics Committee approval, a meeting was held with the mental health manager, ward manager and consultant psychiatrist responsible for the study ward. At this meeting, the study's aims, objectives and methods were explained and fieldwork dates agreed.

Some problems were encountered in securing participation, and it was not possible to proceed in a number of the sites initially selected. The reasons for non-participation were as follows:

- At one site, the Local Research Ethics Committee refused to give approval.
- At another hospital, the principal consultant psychiatrist refused permission because he felt that patient confidentiality might be compromised.
- Finally, the mental health manager at a third site reversed an initial agreement to participate in the study owing to an impending service reorganisation.

Replacement sites were therefore selected, as described above.

There were also some difficulties in securing Local Research Ethics Committee approval in a number of the participating sites. The reasons were:

- concern about whether patient confidentiality would be preserved;
- some misunderstanding of qualitative research methods;
- concern about the extent of disruption in busy acute wards.

It was only after elaborate negotiations that approval was eventually granted.

These delays substantially disrupted the original fieldwork timetable.

Statistical profile of fieldwork sites

The purpose of compiling a service profile for each site was to locate and contextualise each within its respective service system. Four sets of data were sought.

Local services. The mental health manager was asked to complete a Trust Profile Questionnaire (see Appendix 2) for local mental health services, including community services. Only 27% (3) of the questionnaires were completed and returned.

Ward. The ward manager was asked to complete a Ward Environment Questionnaire (see Appendix 3) about ward facilities, and a Ward Manager Questionnaire (see Appendix 4) about the operational routines and therapeutic practices employed. In the case of both questionnaires, 91% (10) were completed and returned.

Staffing. The mental health manager was asked to supply details of staff in post during March 1989 and March 1994 or 1995, so that differences in the workforce profiles between the two dates, in terms of number on duty, grades and qualifications, could be identified.

Obtaining data for 1989 proved difficult. Only two sites (18%) were able to provide some of the staff data (and the Department of Health were unable to help). With respect to 1994 or 1995 data, some data were obtained from all sites, but only two sites (18%) were able to make a full response. The principal gaps in the data were sickness levels among staff for 1989 and 1994 or 1995, and the number and grade of staff in post for 1989.

Patients. The mental health manager was also asked to provide details of ward patients during March 1989 and March 1994 or 1995 in order to identify differences in the patient population between the two dates.

Again, obtaining data for 1989 proved difficult, and again, no site was able to provide all patient data. With respect to 1994 or 1995 data, some data were obtained from all sites, but only two sites (18%) were able to respond fully. Key missing data included the gender and ethnic minority compositions of ward patients, medical diagnoses of patients and details about admissions to, and discharges from, the ward.

It proved impossible, therefore, to compile a comprehensive service profile over time for any of the fieldwork sites. The principal reason given by mental health managers for the data gaps was that, following the 1991 health service reforms and the creation of NHS Trusts, no local facility archived these data. Therefore, to obtain such data would involve too much administrative staff time compiling the relevant information from a number of sources. Owing to the absence of some data, the research team and members of the Research Advisory Group (RAG) accepted that the level of response was in some cases too small to provide meaningful comparisons.

Pre-pilot and pilot studies

Pre-pilot studies were carried out before starting the interviews and observations of nurses and patients at the fieldwork sites. Pre-piloting helped to develop:

- interview schedules (see Appendix 6);
- observation sheets (see Appendix 7).

The pre-pilots also contributed to the development of a feasible fieldwork project plan (see Appendix 5) and were undertaken in two hospitals not involved in the main study – a Water Tower and a general hospital – in sites in the former Yorkshire RHA. Trial interviews were undertaken with four nurses in the Water Tower hospital and two in the general hospital. Additionally, six patients in the Water Tower hospital and five in the general hospital were interviewed. Appendix 8 summarises the issues raised during the pre-pilots, which provided the basis for the interview schedules used with nurses and patients during the main study.

The purpose of the main pilot study was threefold:

1. to test the fieldwork procedures;
2. to test the research instruments;
3. to develop an approach to analysing interview transcripts.

The pilot study was undertaken in the general hospital used for the pre-pilot study. Interviews were conducted with 5 patients, and with 13 ward staff of the following grades: 2 Fs, 3 Es, 3 Ds and 5 As. Piloting showed that the overall project plan was feasible. The full report of the pilot studies is contained in Appendix 9.

As a result of the experiences gained during the pre-pilot and pilot studies, the research instruments were refined and an overall fieldwork plan agreed by the RAG (see Appendix 5).

Main study

Individual interviews were carried out over 6 days from Sunday to Friday, using the interview schedules developed during the pre-pilot and pilot studies. Eighty-five per cent of the interviews were audio-taped and later transcribed. At each site, the following procedures were followed when undertaking interviews of ward staff and patients.

A list of patients, excluding those on leave from the ward and those considered too ill to participate in the study, was provided by the ward manager. The remaining patients were randomly selected by the researchers and approached until five agreed to participate in the study. At interview, patients were asked to complete a Patient Profile Questionnaire about their current admission, referral and living circumstances prior to admission. Fifty-one questionnaires (98%) were completed (see Appendix 10).

Additionally, ward managers were asked to provide details about the staff duty rota during the fieldwork period. These data enabled the researchers to prepare a timetable for interviewing ward staff. All grades of ward staff were interviewed about the nursing care provided to patients, as was the ward manager, who was also asked additional questions about ward routines and practices (see Appendix 4).

At interview, ward staff were asked to complete a Nurse Activity and Personal Details Questionnaire about activities they carried out for and with patients, and information about themselves such as qualifications and grade. One hundred and ten (93%) were completed (see Appendix 11). Staff who had been in post for 5 years or more were asked to compare their present workload with their workload 5 years before. In addition, the named nurses for the five patients who participated in the study were asked about the care they provided for those patients.

In contrast to the difficulty in obtaining data from mental health managers at fieldwork sites, no ward staff at any site refused to participate in the study. As many as possible of the staff on duty during the week of fieldwork were interviewed. In practice, approximately 80% of staff at each participating site were interviewed. Individual interviews were held with 118 members of staff with the following grades:

- 1 H
- 11 Gs
- 14 Fs
- 41 Es
- 22 Ds
- 1 B
- 28 A grade nursing assistants.

In addition, 52 patients were interviewed about their illnesses and how their days in hospital were occupied (see Chapter 4 for details).

Non-participant observation of ward staff and patients

Nurses and patients were also observed over an extended period both to validate what they reported at interview and to give an indication of the range of activities in which staff and patients might be involved during a typical week. Two types of observation were undertaken and used in the report:

- recorded observations of three shifts at each fieldwork site;
- perceptions of the two researchers who carried out the fieldwork at each site.

The activity analysis list used for ward staff and patients during recorded observation periods was that used in previous studies undertaken by the Nuffield Institute for Health (Hurst, 1995a). A former mental health nurse, who had undertaken observational work in previous nursing studies, acted as non-participant observer. The activities of all the ward staff and the five participating patients were recorded at all sites every 15 minutes during three shifts (see Appendix 7): early, late and night shift. This involved the nurse researcher systematically walking around the ward to observe what principal activity was being undertaken by ward staff and patients. If it was not readily apparent to the nurse researcher what activity was being undertaken, he or she would ask the member of staff or patient to explain at the time or, if that was not convenient, soon after the event.

Initially, there were difficulties in undertaking these recorded observations. Anxious ward staff needed to be reassured about their purpose. Some felt that they were involved in time-and-motion studies, which recorded the time taken by them to undertake different activities. However, after reassurance, all staff agreed to be studied.

The range of activities recorded was categorised under four headings:

1. *Direct patient care*: one-to-one contact between a member of staff and patient, for example: discussions about an aspect of patient care, care planning, assessment, comforting or controlling a patient and crisis intervention; group sessions in the ward; staff dispensing medication to patients; observations of patients by staff; staff assisting patients with their personal care; staff accompanying a patient going for treatment off the ward; staff undertaking recreation activities with a patient or group of patients; and members of staff who assisted with ECT.
2. *Indirect patient care*: discussions between hospital staff and others about a particular patient, for example: attending the MDT meeting (ward round); shift hand-over periods; and a member of staff speaking to a particular patient's relatives.
3. *Associated work*: work that might not be directly related to patient care but is nevertheless important for the effective delivery of nursing care, for example: meetings of ward staff and doctors, other professionals or other ward staff; undertaking office duties; teaching student nurses; carrying out domestic duties; undertaking duties off the ward; and completing errands.
4. *Personal time*: staff breaks during shifts as well as unoccupied staff.

Chapters 5 and 6 provide a detailed discussion of the observational data obtained and a comparison of the findings with previous data collected over the period 1985–93 (Hurst, 1995a).

Additionally, notes were taken by one of the researchers as he or she observed MDT meetings (ward round), and a number of shift hand-over periods, to record the type of information shared with colleagues and to examine the nursing role in such forums (see Chapter 6).

Researcher perceptions

The value of using researcher perceptions of fieldwork sites is that formal recorded observations are unable adequately to portray the context in which nursing staff were working, that is, how busy wards were and the pressures on nurses. Nurse observers were also able to obtain some impression of how typical the periods observed were of activity in the ward. For example, owing to 15 minute snapshots, few observations were recorded of staff involvement in crisis intervention in the ward. However, the researchers were aware of such occurrences during the course of the fieldwork at several sites and could record the impact upon work within the ward.

Furthermore, researchers often waited in the ward office and were able to observe and record how nursing staff used the ward office. This could be, for example, whether conversations were about patients or personal issues; whether nurses were completing paperwork; whether they were using the ward office as a sanctuary from other ward activities; and whether patients were allowed into the office freely, or whether the office door appeared to be used as a barrier between staff and patients.

Analysing fieldwork data

Four rich and extensive data sets were collected from all sites:

- statistical profiles;
- staff and patient interviews;
- staff and patient questionnaires;
- non-participant observations.

The latter three data sets were analysed site by site on the basis of staff grade, patient type, region, hospital type and bed occupancy level. The results are set out fully in Chapters 4, 5 and 6. Data about staff activity were compared with Hurst's similar data collected over the period 1985–93. This allowed the research team to identify trends illustrating the changing nature of psychiatric nursing.

Nurse and patient interview data were analysed using the Ethnograph software package. The data from the Nurse Activity and Personal Details Questionnaire, and from the Patient Profile Questionnaire for patients (see above), were analysed using the Statistical Package for Social Sciences in order to map similarities and differences across sites. Observation data were analysed in a similar way to these questionnaire data.

In total, these analyses triangulated information about the range of activities that each grade of staff undertook during the three observed shifts and enabled comparisons to be made across sites and over time using Hurst's data (1995a).

Postal survey

A postal survey was undertaken in a number of former RHAs, the purpose of which was to obtain an overview of ward organisation, management, the deployment of nurses and the nature of patient populations in acute psychiatric settings, thus complementing the surveys of nurses and patients at the fieldwork sites.

The approach adopted was that used in a previous nursing study carried out by the Nuffield Institute for Health, in which an 80% response rate had been achieved (Southwell *et al.*, 1993).

First, the regional co-ordinator with responsibility for mental health services within two of the former RHAs was contacted for the names and addresses of all mental health managers with responsibilities for acute services in his or her region.

After securing the mental health managers' agreements to participate in the study, each was each sent a copy of the Trust Profile Questionnaire. The questionnaire asked for information about mental health hospital and community services available in each manager's area (see Appendix 12). Additionally, each was sent a number of copies of the Ward Profile and Operational Routines for Acute Psychiatric Admission Wards Questionnaire (see Appendix 13). These questionnaires were to be completed by all ward managers (G grade nurses) who were responsible for an acute psychiatric ward, and asked for information about ward staff and patients. Freepost envelopes were supplied for the return of the questionnaires.

Finally, each mental health manager was asked to complete a reply slip with the following details:

- name of the hospital;
- names and telephone numbers of acute psychiatric admission wards;
- names and contact numbers of all ward managers.

Non-respondents were contacted 1 month after posting the questionnaire.

Postal surveys were carried out in two former RHAs: Wessex and South Western. These were chosen partly to balance the northern emphasis of fieldwork sites, but mainly because they met the criteria used for selecting other sites. The former Wessex RHA showed similarities to the former Northern RHA, and the former South Western RHA showed similarities to the former Yorkshire RHA (see Appendix 1). Thirteen Trust Profile Questionnaires were sent to mental health managers, and 42 Ward Profile and Operational Routines for Acute Psychiatric Admission Wards Questionnaires were sent to ward managers in these two former regions.

Response rates were very low despite two follow-up letters and numerous phone calls:

- 8% (1) of the mental health manager questionnaires were completed and returned.
- 21% (9) of the ward manager questionnaires were completed and returned. However, 12% (5) originated from the same hospital.

The main reason cited by mental health managers for non-completion of questionnaires was pressure of work and an excessive volume of paperwork. This response rate was disappointing, especially in view of the 80% return achieved in the previous Nuffield Institute for Health study using an identical approach and seeking similar data. It was agreed by the RAG that the number of responses was too small to yield valid and reliable data.

Feedback seminars for fieldwork sites

More successful, however, were the two seminars held for representatives, including managers, educationists and clinicians from fieldwork sites. The purpose of the seminars was threefold:

1. to provide staff from participating sites with a summary of findings (Higgins *et al.*, 1996a, 1996b, 1996c);
2. to test the utility and validity of the findings;
3. to begin formulating recommendations.

The first seminar was for sites in Regions A and B, which 36 representatives from those sites attended. The second was for sites in Region C, from which eight representatives attended (Higgins *et al.*, 1996d, 1996e).

After a brief presentation of findings, participants were divided into groups of approximately 4–6 and asked to consider the following questions:

- To what extent were the findings an accurate reflection of nursing work?
- What were the implications of the findings for mental health services?

- What key messages should be conveyed to the Department of Health?

Appendix 14 summarises the issues raised at the two seminars. The seminars were invaluable for formulating the study's overall findings, conclusions and recommendations (discussed in Chapter 7).

Summary

- The selection of regions and fieldwork sites was based upon an analysis of various data and the Research Advisory Group members' knowledge of mental health services.
- The study was carried out in the former RHAs of Yorkshire and Northern, and at sites in Inner London. Fieldwork sites comprised a variety of locations and hospital types.
- Some problems were encountered in securing site participation and in obtaining data from all sites. Even so, 118 members of ward staff and 52 patients participated in the study in 11 sites.
- The postal survey yielded a poor response, one too small to provide useful data.
- Two feedback seminars were held for fieldwork sites in Regions A and B, and Region C, respectively.

Chapter 4
The hospital care context

The ward environments and patient populations in the 11 fieldwork sites are discussed using the data described in Chapter 3:

- nurse and patient interview material;
- recorded observations of nurses and patients;
- researcher perceptions;
- ward environment and ward manager questionnaires.

Ward managers were asked how typical were conditions in the ward during the fieldwork week. At sites A2, A3, A4, B5 and B6, wards were reported to be quieter than usual. At sites A1, B7, B8, C9, C10 and C11, wards were described as typical.

Chapter 3 revealed that it was impossible to provide a detailed account of how wards sat within local service systems or to identify whether staff and patient profiles had changed between 1989 and 1995. However, much can still be said about the context of care at fieldwork sites using two case studies that illustrate differences between sites. First, however, an overview of ward environments is provided.

Ward environments

An analysis of Ward Environment Questionnaires and researcher perceptions revealed that the age, type and location of hospitals, the shape and size of wards, and the types of patient accommodation were different (Tables 4.1 and 4.2; see also Higgins *et al.*, 1995a, 1995b).

Table 4.1 Fieldwork sites

Site	Hospital type	Period built	Location	Bed complement
A1	3	1970s–90s	A	28
A2	1	1940s–60s	D	23
A3	2	1850s–1900s	D	22
A4	3	1850s–1900s	C	26
B5	3	1910s–30s	C	9 (+5)
B6	2	1850s–1900s	B	28
B7	1	1970s–90s	A	16
B8	1	1970s–90s	B	25
C9	1	1970s–90s	A	17
C10	3	1910s–30s	A	25
C11	2	1850s–1900s	A	22

Type: 1 = district general hospital; 2 = Water Tower hospital; 3 = other service settings. Location: A = inner city; B = rural; C = urban; D = rural, near large town/city.

Note: B5: for patients who required more secure accommodation, staff had access to five beds in a traditional Water Tower hospital located 6 miles away.

Table 4.2 Ward characteristics

Site	A	B	C	D	E	F	G	H	I	J	K	L	M	N	O	P
A1	1	1	1	1	1	2	1	1	8	5	1	1	1	3	1	1
A2	1	1	1	1	2	2	1	2	8	5	1	1	1	1	1	1
A3	1	1	1	1	1	2	1	2	4	3	1	1	2	3	1	2
A4	1	1	1	1	2	2	1	2	8	4	2	1	3	3	1	3
B5	1	1	1	1	3	1	1	1	3	4	1	1	3	3	2	3
B6	1	1	1	1	1	1	1	2	6	4	2	1	1	3	1	1
B7	1	1	1	1	2	1	1	2	2	2	2	1	2	1	1	1
B8	1	1	1	1	3	1	1	2	4	7	1	1	1	2	1	1
C9	1	1	1	1	3	1	1	2	4	4	1	1	1	3	1	2
C10	1	2	1	1	2	2	1	2	6	4	1	1	2	3	2	2
C11	1	1	1	1	1	2	1	2	6	4	2	1	1	2	1	2

A: 1 = all beds with bedside lights.

B: 1 = strip lighting throughout the ward; 2 = some strip lighting in the ward.

C: 1 = all windows curtained.

D: 1 = all beds with curtains.

E: 1 = patient accommodation consisted primarily of single-sex dormitories; 2 = patient accommodation consisted primarily of single-sex bays; 3 = patient accommodation consisted primarily of individual rooms.

F: 1 = all floors were carpeted; 2 = all floors carpeted, except corridors.

G: 1 = telephones with an audible ring at night.

H: 1 = ward heating was under the control of staff; 2 = ward heating was not under the control of staff.

(contd)

Table 4.2 (contd)

I: Number of toilets.

J: Number of baths/showers.

K: 1 = all beds fitted with buzzers; 2 = most beds fitted with buzzers.

L: 1 = ward office was located away from sleeping areas.

M: 1 = ward was located at ground level; 2 = ward was located above ground level; 3 = ward was on a split-level, located on at least two floors.

N: 1 = smoking was allowed in the day room at any time; 2 = a smoking room was provided for patients; 3 = smoking was not allowed.

O: 1 = written information about ward routines was provided to patients on admission; 2 = oral information about ward routines was provided to patients on admission.

P: 1 = group activities were organised by therapists in the hospital's occupational therapy department; 2 = group activities were organised by therapists and nursing staff in the ward; 3 = group activities were organised by nursing staff in the ward.

Summary of the features of fieldwork sites

Hospital type

Three types of hospital settings were included in the study:

- district general hospitals (four): A2, B7, B8 and C9;
- Water Tower psychiatric hospitals (three): A3, B6 and C11;
- other service settings (four): A1 was a ward in a purpose built mental health unit; A4 was a ward in a former elderly care hospital; B5 was a community unit in a converted house; and C10 was a ward in a former general hospital. Sites A1 and C10 also housed general acute wards and outpatient and therapy services.

Period built

The approximate building period for each hospital was:
- 1850s–1900s (four): A3, A4, B6 and C11;
- 1910s–30s (two): B5 and C10;
- 1940s–60s (one): A2;
- 1970s–90s (four): A1, B7, B8 and C9.

Location

Hospitals were situated in a variety of geographical locations:

- deprived inner-city areas (five): A1, B7, C9, C10 and C11;
- other urban settings (two): A4 and B5;
- rural, some distance from an urban centre (two): B6 and B8;
- rural, but close to a major urban centre (two): A2 and A3.

Bed complement

The bed complement of fieldwork sites ranged from:

- fewer than 20 beds (three): B5, B7 and C9;
- between 21 and 25 beds (five): A2, A3, B8, C10 and C11;
- 26 beds or more (three): A1, A4 and B6.

Summary of the ward characteristics

Patient accommodation

Three main types of patient accommodation were included in the study:

1. single-sex dormitories (four): A1, A3, B6 and C11;
2. single-sex bays (four): A2, A4, B7 and C10;
3. individual rooms (three): B5, B8 and C9.

Ward layout and design

The similarities and differences of ward layout and design are described below. The following features were common to most sites (exceptions being indicated):

- All beds had individual bedside lights.
- Fluorescent strip lighting was used throughout the ward (except in site C10).
- All windows were curtained.
- All beds had their own curtains.
- Telephones had an audible ring at night.
- The ward office was situated away from sleeping areas.
- Smoking was not allowed in the ward (except A2 and B7 where smoking was allowed in the day room, and B8 and C11 where a separate smoking room was provided).
- Ward heating was not controlled by staff (except sites A1 and B5).
- Written information about ward routines was provided to all patients on admission (except B5 and C10, where only oral information was provided).

The following features highlighted differences between sites:

- At five sites, all floors were carpeted: B5, B6, B7, B8 and C9; and at six sites most floors were carpeted, except corridors: A1, A2, A3, A4, C10 and C11.

- At seven sites, all beds were fitted with buzzers: A1, A2, A3, B5, B8, C9 and C10; and at four sites, not all beds were fitted with buzzers: A4, B6, B7 and C11.
- At five sites, the ward was located at ground level: A1, A2, B6, B8 and C11; at four sites, the ward was located above ground level: A3, B7, C9 and C10; and at two sites, the ward was split between at least two floors: A4 and B5.

Patient populations

All sites cared for patients classified as suffering from a functional mental illness. Patients classified as suffering from an organic condition – generally older people with dementia – were usually cared for in the care of the elderly wards. Staff at each site reported that patient profiles during the fieldwork week were representative of the patient population.

In this chapter, patient populations are discussed by region, geographical location of hospital, hospital type and bed occupancies, using data from interviews, observations and ward manager questionnaires (Tables 4.3A–D and 4.4A–D below; see also Higgins *et al.*, 1995a, 1995b).

Features of patient populations

Bed occupancy

Three categories were identified:

1. sites operating at 85% occupancy or less (85% being the Royal College of Psychiatrists recommended maximum level at which wards should operate): A3 and A4;
2. sites operating at between 86% and 99%: A2, B6, B7 and B8;
3. sites operating at 100% or above: A1, B5, C9, C10 and C11.

A number of strategies were employed to deal with wards above 100% occupancy:

- Additional beds were provided in the ward.
- Patients were cared for in other wards or in other hospitals.
- Patients were housed in the private sector as extra contractual referrals (ECRs), particularly at Region C sites.
- Patients were granted extended leave (particularly at Region C sites).

Whichever strategy was employed, wards were still overcrowded because patients housed elsewhere usually came into the ward during the day for meals or treatment, or to participate in group activities (see also Audit Commission, 1994; Faulkner *et al.*, 1994; House of Commons Health Committee, 1994; Mental Health Foundation, 1994; Mental Health Task Force, 1994; Mental Health Act Commission, 1995; Powell *et al.*, 1995).

The main bed occupancy features were:

- *Region.* All regions had average bed occupancies above that recommended by the Royal College of Psychiatrists: Region C had levels in excess of 100%, and all but two sites – A1 and B5 – in Regions A and B had levels below 100% (Table 4.3A). Representatives from some of those sites at the feedback seminar for Regions A and B said that acute wards had consistently operated at or above 100% occupancy since the fieldwork had been completed.
- *Geographical location.* Inner-city sites A1, B7, C9, C10 and C11 – all except B7 – had occupancies in excess of 100%, and only one site from the other locations – B5 – had an occupancy of 100% (Tables 4.3B and 4.3D).
- *Hospital type.* District general hospital sites – A2, B7, B8 and C9 – had average occupancies over 100%, and Water Tower hospitals and other service settings both had 98% occupancies (see Table 4.3C). However, average figures were skewed by the high occupancy levels of Region C sites compared with other sites.

Table 4.3A Patient populations by region (A versus B versus C)

Site	Bed occupancy (%)	Sex (male: female)	Average age (standard deviation)	Patients known to staff (%)	Average length of stay (weeks) Reported	Actual	Ethnic minority (%)
A1	107	12:18	38 (12.5)	96	4–8	6.6	32
A2	96	16:6	36 (15.7)	82	4–8	12.0	0
A3	73	7:9	43 (16.9)	75	4–8	2.6	0
A4	73	15:4	47 (18.1)	79	<4	3.2	0
Average	87	13:9	41 (15.8)	83		6.1	8
B5	100	2:7	36 (13.8)	55	4–8	7.0	0

(contd)

Table 4.3A (contd)

Site	Bed occupancy (%)	Sex (male: female)	Average age (standard deviation)	Patients known to staff (%)	Average length of stay (weeks) Reported	Actual	Ethnic minority (%)
B6	86	15:9	44 (20.4)	83	4–8	3.5	0
B7	94	10:5	39 (15.8)	88	4–8	2.5	7
B8	88	8:14	42 (14.6)	73	4–8	41.7	0
Average	**92**	**9:9**	**40 (16.2)**	**75**		**4.3 – B8** **13.7 + B8**	**2**
C9	153	17:9	31 (9.2)	92	4–8	5.6	55
C10	112	8:18	43 (13.2)	83	6–10	9.2	34
C11	136	21:9	44 (12.8)	85	2–8	9.5	43
Average	**134**	**15:12**	**39 (11.7)**	**86**		**8.1**	**44**

Notes: Average length of stay (weeks): the reported figure refers to the approximate range in weeks ward managers said that patients stayed in the ward; and the actual figures refers to the average length of stay of patients –usually five–who participated in the study at each site.

B8: Two figures are provided for the actual average length of stay: with (+) and without (–) the site. One of the patients interviewed had been in hospital for over a year and thus skewed the figure for the site.

Ethnic minority (%): refers to patients that were not classified as White British, including: Black Afro-Caribbean; Black Asian: Indian, Pakistani and Bangladeshi; and Other White: German, Irish and Spanish. Patients in the latter category were primarily located in Region C sites.

Table 4.3B Patient populations by geographical location of hospital (inner city versus other urban versus rural)

Site	Bed occupancy (%)	Sex (male: female)	Average age (standard deviation)	Patients known to staff (%)	Average length of stay (weeks) Reported	Actual	Ethnic minority (%)
A1	107	12:18	38 (12.5)	96	4–8	6.6	32
B7	94	10:5	39 (15.8)	88	4–8	2.5	7

(contd)

Table 4.3B (contd)

Site	Bed occupancy (%)	Sex (male: female)	Average age (standard deviation)	Patients known to staff (%)	Average length of stay (weeks) Reported	Actual	Ethnic minority (%)
C9	153	17:9	31 (9.2)	92	4–8	5.6	55
C10	112	8:18	43 (13.2)	83	6–10	9.2	34
C11	136	21:9	44 (12.8)	85	2–8	9.5	43
Average	**120**	**14:12**	**39 (12.7)**	**89**		**6.7**	**34**
A4	73	15:4	47 (18.1)	79	<4	3.2	0
B5	100	2:7	36 (13.8)	55	4–8	7.0	0
Average	**87**	**9:6**	**42 (16.0)**	**67**		**5.1**	**0**
A2	96	16:6	36 (15.7)	82	4–8	12.0	0
A3	73	7:9	43 (16.9)	75	4–8	2.6	0
B6	86	15:9	44 (20.4)	83	4–8	3.5	0
B8	88	8:14	42) (14.6)	73	4–8	41.7	0
Average	**86**	**12:10**	**41 (16.9)**	**78**		**6.0 – B8 15.0 + B8**	**0**

Table 4.3C Patient populations by hospital type (district general versus Water Tower versus other service settings)

Site	Bed occupancy (%)	Sex (male: female)	Average age (standard deviation)	Patients known to staff (%)	Average length of stay (weeks) Reported	Actual	Ethnic minority (%)
A2	96	16:6	36 (15.7)	82	4–8	12.0	0
B7	94	10:5	39) (15.8	88	4–8	2.5	7
B8	88	8:14	42 (14.6)	73	4–8	41.7	0

(contd)

Table 4.3C (contd)

Site	Bed occupancy (%)	Sex (male: female)	Average age (standard deviation)	Patients known to staff (%)	Average length of stay (weeks) Reported	Actual	Ethnic minority (%)
C9	153	17:9	31 (9.2)	92	4–8	5.6	55
Average	**108**	**13:9**	**37 (13.8)**	**84**		**6.7 – B8 15.5 + B8**	**16**
A3	73	7:9	43 (16.8)	75	4–8	2.6	0
B6	86	15:9	44 (20.4)	83	4–8	3.5	0
C11	136	21:9	44 (12.8)	85	2–8	9.5	43
Average	**98**	**14:9**	**44 (16.7)**	**81**		**5.2**	**14**
A1	107	12:18	38 (12.5)	96	4–8	6.6	32
A4	73	15:4	47 (18.1)	79	<4	3.2	0
B5	100	2:7	36 (13.8)	55	4–8	7.0	0
C10	112	8:18	43 (13.2)	83	6–10	9.2	34
Average	**98**	**9:12**	**41 (14.4)**	**78**		**6.5**	**17**

Table 4.3D Patient populations by bed occupancy level (≥ 100% versus < 100%)

Site	Bed occupancy (%)	Sex (male: female)	Average age (standard deviation)	Patients known to staff (%)	Average length of stay (weeks) Reported	Actual	Ethnic minority (%)
A1	107	12:18	38 (12.5)	96	4–8	6.6	32
B5	100	2:7	36 (13.8)	55	4–8	7.0	0
C9	153	17:9	31 (9.2)	92	4–8	5.6	55
C10	112	8:18	43 (13.2)	83	6–10	9.2	34
C11	136	21:9	44 (12.8)	85	2–8	9.5	43

(contd)

Table 4.3D (contd)

Site	Bed occupancy (%)	Sex (male: female)	Average age (standard deviation)	Patients known to staff (%)	Average length of stay (weeks) Reported	Actual	Ethnic minority (%)
Average	122	12:12	38 (12.3)	82		7.6	33
A2	96	16:6	36 (15.7)	82	4–8	12.0	0
A3	73	7:9	43 (16.9)	75	4–8	2.6	0
A4	73	15:4	47 (18.1)	79	<4	3.2	0
B6	86	15:9	44 (20.4)	83	4–8	3.5	0
B7	94	10:5	39 (15.8)	88	4–8	2.5	7
B8	88	8:14	42 (14.6)	73	4–8	41.7	0
Average	85	12:8	42 (16.9)	80		**4.8 – B8** **10.9 + B8**	1

Male-to-female patient ratio

The key features of the male-to-female patient ratio were as follows:

- There were no significant regional, geographical location of hospital, hospital type or bed occupancy patterns across sites (see Tables 4.3A–D respectively).
- There was roughly an even split between sites where male patients formed the majority – A2, A4, B6, B7, C9 and C11 – and those where female patients were more prevalent – A1, A3, B5, B8 and C10.
- However, average male-to-female ratios revealed a slightly higher proportion of men to women patients in the study wards.

Age of patients

The main characteristics of patients' ages were:

- *Region.* On average, patients in Region C were younger than their counterparts in Regions A and B (see Table 4.3A).

- *Geographical.* On average, patients in hospitals located in inner-city areas – A1, B7, C9, C10 and C11 – were younger than patients located in hospitals in other areas (see Table 4.3B).
- *Hospital type.* Patients in district general hospital sites were on average younger than those located in other hospital settings, and patients located in Water Tower hospitals were on average significantly older than those located in other hospital types (see Table 4.3C).
- *Bed occupancy.* Patients in wards with 100% or more bed occupancy – A1, B5, C9, C10 and C11 – were on average younger than those with a less than 100% occupancy level (see Table 4.3D). (Most wards with 100% or over bed occupancy were located in inner-city areas: A1, C9, C10 and C11.)

Patients with previous admissions

The most significant features of patients known to ward staff are outlined below.

There were no significant regional, location of hospital, hospital type or bed occupancy differences across sites. The most notable characteristic was the high percentage of patients known to staff: except at B5, staff reported that over 70% of inpatients were known to them; and at seven sites – A1, A2, B6, B7, C9, C10 and C11 – the figure was over 80% (see Tables 4.3A–D). Two principal explanations were cited:

- Many patients had been admitted for non-compliance with their medication.
- In a small number of cases, admission had resulted from loss of contact with community services. This meant a revolving door phenomenon for some patients (regular admissions between varying lengths of time in the community), confirming the finding of other recent studies: Audit Commission (1994), House of Commons Health Committee (1994), Powell *et al.* (1995), Lelliot *et al.* (1996).

Staff reported that the 20–30% of patients for whom it was a first admission were often more severely ill than hitherto, and therefore more demanding on nurses' time, and some of those patients already known to staff had become increasingly unpredictable in behaviour. Drug and alcohol abuse were often said to be factors in patients' unpredictable behaviour (the so-called dual diagnosis phenomena).

Consequently, nurses felt that it was sometimes difficult to maintain a safe therapeutic environment in the ward (see Tables 4.4A–D).

Length of inpatient stay

Key features of inpatient stay were:

- *Region.* Region B – with the exception of B8 – had the shortest average length of stay, and Region C had the longest (see Table 4.3A).
- *Geographical location.* Inner-city sites had longer average stays compared with sites in other locations (see Table 4.3B).
- *Hospital type.* Water Tower hospitals had the shortest stays compared with other hospital types (see Table 4.3C).
- *Bed occupancy.* Except B5, sites with the highest occupancy levels were located in inner-city areas (see Table 4.3D).

Ethnic minority patients

The main ethnic characteristics were:

- *Region.* Except for A1, Regions A and B had few patients from an ethnic minority group, and Region C had a high proportion of such patients (see Table 4.3A). The inner-city location of Region C sites accounts for these differences.
- *Geographical location.* Inner-city sites had an average of 34% of patients from ethnic minority groups, and sites in other localities had no patients from these groups (see Table 4.3B).
- *Hospital type.* There were no significant variations (see Table 4.3C).
- *Bed occupancy.* Sites with levels of 100% or over had a high proportion of people from ethnic minority groups, and sites with levels below 100% had no patients from such groups (see Table 4.3D). The urban location of the former sites, and rural location of the latter sites, largely accounts for the difference in occupancy.

Severity of patients' illness

Four indicators were used by ward staff to identify the most severely ill patients (see Tables 4.4A–D):

1. *Dependency.* Patients with a level of 2 or more required some help with daily activities.

2. *Detained patients.* The most severely ill patients were often those who had been compulsorily admitted under a Section of the 1983 Mental Health Act.
3. *Observation level.* Patients placed on level 1 observation were those who were considered to be a potential risk to themselves or to others.
4. Patients diagnosed with *schizophrenia* or *other psychoses* were considered the most unpredictable in terms of mood and behaviour, and were often responsible for many of the crisis intervention activities undertaken by staff.

The principal characteristics of severely ill patients in wards were:

- *Region.* Region C cared for the most severely ill patients: dependency level 2 or more, 76%; detained patients, 44%; observation level 1, 8%; and patients diagnosed with schizophrenia or other psychoses, 77%. The following are the corresponding figures for Regions A and B respectively: dependency level, 47% and 38%; detained patients, 35% and 45%; observation level 1, 1% and 3%; and schizophrenia and other psychoses, 46% and 38% (Table 4.4A).
- *Geographical location.* Inner-city sites had the most severely ill patients, and sites in rural locations the least (Table 4.4B).
- *Hospital type.* Traditional Water Tower hospitals had the least severely ill patients compared with sites located in other service settings (Table 4.4C).
- *Bed occupancy.* Sites with 100% or more occupancy had the most severely ill patients compared with sites with less than 100% occupancy (Table 4.4D). The inner-city location of most of the former sites is worth noting.

Discussion

Ward environments

There were many differences in ward environment between sites (see Tables 4.1 and 4.2). Staff and patients identified features of the environment that were not conducive to patient recovery.

Sites located in old buildings – A2, A3, A4, B6, C10 and 11. The layouts, often similar to those of Nightingale-type wards, or the physical fabric of the wards, were said to be poor for patient recovery. High ceilings and large communal and sleeping areas were common at these sites, exacerbating the noise generated in the wards. Patients frequently commented on the lack of privacy.

Table 4.4A Patients' Illnesses by Region (A versus B versus C)

Site	Dependency level (%)				Detained (%)	Observation level (%)			Medical diagnoses of patients						
	1	2	3	4		1	2	3	Schizophrenia (%)	Other psychoses (%)	Depressive illness (%)	Anxiety condition (%)	Personality disorder (%)	Drug/alcohol/substance misuse (%)	Other (%)
A1	0	86	7	7	57	0	70	30	43	18	18	0	18	0	4
A2	55	32	14	0	41	0	18	82	14	24	52	5	5	5	0
A3	86	6	0	6	19	0	0	100	0	31	31	25	0	13	0
A4	68	21	11	0	21	5	5	90	16	37	16	32	0	0	0
Average	**52**	**36**	**8**	**3**	**35**	**1**	**23**	**76**	**18**	**28**	**29**	**16**	**6**	**5**	**1**
B5	67	22	11	0	88	0	11	88	55	11	0	0	22	0	11
B6	46	46	8	0	25	4	8	88	8	13	26	17	4	33	0
B7	73	13	13	0	47	7	0	93	33	7	27	7	7	14	7
B8	59	32	9	0	18	0	5	95	9	18	55	0	5	5	10
Average	**61**	**28**	**10**	**0**	**45**	**3**	**6**	**91**	**26**	**12**	**27**	**6**	**10**	**13**	**7**
C9	39	50	8	4	54	12	12	76	81	13	6	0	0	0	0
C10	4	85	12	0	39	4	14	82	46	19	23	0	4	0	8
C11	30	60	7	3	43	7	23	70	50	23	20	0	0	0	7
Average	**24**	**65**	**9**	**2**	**44**	**8**	**16**	**76**	**59**	**18**	**16**	**0**	**1**	**0**	**5**

Table 4.4B Patients' illnesses by geographical location of hospitals (inner city versus other urban versus rural)

Site	Dependency level (%)				Detained (%)	Observation level (%)			Schizophrenia (%)	Other psychoses (%)	Medical diagnoses of patients				
											Depressive illness (%)	Anxiety condition (%)	Personality disorder (%)	Drug/alcohol/substance misuse (%)	Other (%)
	1	2	3	4		1	2	3							
A1	0	86	7	7	57	0	70	30	43	18	18	0	18	0	4
B7	73	13	13	0	47	7	0	93	33	7	27	7	7	14	7
C9	39	50	8	4	54	12	12	76	81	13	6	0	0	0	0
C10	4	85	12	0	39	4	14	82	46	19	23	0	4	0	8
C11	30	60	7	3	40	7	23	70	50	23	20	0	0	0	7
Average	**29**	**59**	**9**	**3**	**47**	**6**	**24**	**70**	**51**	**16**	**19**	**1**	**6**	**3**	**5**
A4	68	21	11	0	21	5	5	90	16	37	16	32	0	0	0
B5	67	22	11	0	88	0	11	88	55	11	0	0	22	0	11
Average	**68**	**22**	**11**	**0**	**55**	**3**	**8**	**89**	**36**	**24**	**8**	**16**	**11**	**0**	**6**
A2	55	32	14	0	41	0	18	82	14	24	52	5	5	5	0
A3	86	6	0	6	19	0	0	100	0	31	31	25	0	13	0
B6	46	46	8	0	25	4	8	88	8	13	26	17	4	33	0
B8	59	32	9	0	18	0	5	95	9	18	55	0	5	5	10
Average	**62**	**29**	**8**	**2**	**26**	**1**	**8**	**91**	**8**	**22**	**41**	**12**	**4**	**14**	**3**

Table 4.4C Patients' illnesses by hospital type (district general versus Water Tower versus other service settings)

Site	Dependency level (%)				Detained (%)	Observation level (%)			Schizophrenia (%)	Other psychoses (%)	Depressive illness (%)	Anxiety condition (%)	Personality disorder (%)	Drug/alcohol/substance misuse (%)	Other (%)
	1	2	3	4		1	2	3							
A2	55	32	14	0	41	0	18	82	14	24	52	5	5	5	0
B7	73	13	13	0	47	7	0	93	33	7	27	7	7	14	7
B8	59	32	9	0	18	0	5	95	9	18	55	0	5	5	10
C9	39	50	8	4	54	12	12	76	81	13	6	0	0	0	0
Average	**57**	**32**	**11**	**1**	**40**	**5**	**9**	**87**	**34**	**16**	**35**	**3**	**4**	**6**	**4**
A3	86	6	0	6	19	0	0	100	0	31	31	25	0	13	0
B6	46	46	8	0	25	4	8	88	8	13	26	17	4	33	0
C11	30	60	7	3	40	7	23	70	50	23	20	0	0	0	7
Average	**54**	**37**	**5**	**3**	**28**	**4**	**10**	**86**	**19**	**22**	**26**	**14**	**1**	**15**	**2**
A1	0	86	7	7	57	0	70	30	43	18	18	0	18	0	4
A4	68	21	11	0	21	5	5	90	16	37	16	32	0	0	0
B5	67	22	11	0	88	0	11	88	55	11	0	0	22	0	11
C10	4	85	12	0	39	4	14	82	46	19	23	0	4	0	8
Average	**35**	**54**	**10**	**2**	**51**	**2**	**25**	**73**	**40**	**21**	**14**	**8**	**11**	**0**	**6**

Medical diagnoses of patients

Table 4.4D Patients' illnesses by bed occupancy level (≥ 100% versus <100%)

Site	Dependency level (%)				Detained (%)	Observation level (%)			Medical diagnoses of patients						
									Schizophrenia (%)	Other psychoses (%)	Depressive illness (%)	Anxiety condition (%)	Personality disorder (%)	Drug/ alcohol/ substance misuse (%)	Other (%)
	1	2	3	4		1	2	3							
A1	0	86	7	7	57	0	70	30	43	18	18	0	18	0	4
B5	67	22	11	0	88	0	11	88	55	11	0	0	22	0	11
C9	39	50	8	4	54	12	12	76	81	13	6	0	0	0	0
C10	4	85	12	0	39	4	14	82	46	19	23	0	4	0	8
C11	30	60	7	3	40	7	23	70	50	23	20	0	0	0	7
Average	**28**	**61**	**9**	**3**	**56**	**5**	**26**	**69**	**55**	**17**	**13**	**0**	**9**	**0**	**6**
A2	55	32	14	0	41	0	18	82	14	24	52	5	5	5	0
A3	86	6	6	0	19	0	0	100	0	31	31	25	0	13	0
A4	68	21	11	0	21	5	5	90	16	37	16	32	0	0	0
B6	46	46	8	0	25	4	8	88	8	13	26	17	4	33	0
B7	73	13	13	0	47	7	0	93	33	7	27	7	7	14	7
B8	59	32	9	0	18	0	5	95	9	18	55	0	5	5	10
Average	**65**	**25**	**9**	**1**	**29**	**3**	**6**	**91**	**13**	**22**	**35**	**14**	**4**	**12**	**3**

Dependency level (%) refers to nurses' perceptions of the extent to which patients required assistance with walking, eating and drinking, continence and personal care, and the degree of mental health dysfunction, on a scale of 0–5, the latter indicating the greatest level of need.

Detained (%) refers to the percentage of patients compulsorily detained in hospital.

Observation level (%) sites used a 3-point scale as follows. Observation level 1: patients must remain within touching distance of a member of staff at all times; usually reserved for patients who are considered to be a risk to themselves or to others. Observation level 2: patients must remain within sight of a member of staff at all times. Observation level 3: patients can move freely in and out of the ward, but they are encouraged to let a member of staff know if they wish to leave the ward.

Sites located in modern buildings – A1, B5, B7, B8 and C9. The ward layout also created problems for staff. The prevalence of single rooms, welcomed by patients because of the privacy provided, made it difficult for staff to monitor what patients were doing, compared with the traditional, dormitory layout in older buildings. There was a tendency for patients to remain in their rooms and not take part in ward activities. This lack of association with others was considered by many nurses to be detrimental to recovery.

Mixed-sex wards. Patients and staff questioned the merits of mixed-sex wards. Female patients in particular said that they often felt intimidated and threatened by male patients, owing to the aggressive behaviour exhibited by some men suffering from psychotic conditions (see Tables 4.4A–D). This seriously concerned a number of women because physical or sexual abuse by men contributed to their illnesses.

Diversity of needs. All sites cared for a diversity of needs (see Tables 4.3A–D and 4.4A–D), the wisdom of which was questioned by staff. The patient mix in many wards created problems. For example, patients with a depression or anxiety were often distressed by the noise and behaviour exhibited by patients suffering from severe schizophrenia and other psychotic illnesses.

Patient populations

The widely held perception of those working in acute mental health services that they were caring for a more difficult patient population than previously has been corroborated in this study. Moreover, it is possible to distinguish patient populations. Difficult populations – A1, B7, C9, C10 and C11 – had the following combination of characteristics (see Tables 4.3A–D and 4.4A–D):

- high bed occupancy levels;
- generally a location in inner-city areas, irrespective of hospital type;
- a younger patient profile;
- more male patients;
- over 80% of patients being known to staff;
- a high proportion of patients from ethnic minorities;
- on average, patients being in hospital for longer periods of time;
- a severely ill and dependent population.

Manageable populations – A2, A3, A4, B5, B6 and B8 – had the following characteristics (see Tables 4.3A–D and 4.4A–D above):

- lower bed occupancy levels;
- generally a location in suburban or rural locations, especially for Water Tower hospitals;
- an older patient profile;
- more female patients;
- fewer patients known to staff;
- few patients from ethnic minorities;
- on average, patients having shorter periods of time in hospital;
- a less severely ill and less dependent population.

Case studies 4.1 and 4.2 below illustrate the key differences between the two types of patient population: difficult and manageable respectively.

CASE STUDY 4.1

C9 was located in a mental health unit in the grounds of a district general hospital, in a socio-economically deprived area. This area had one of the highest levels of unemployment in the region, particularly among the young Afro-Caribbean males, who comprised a high proportion of the ward's patients. Men outnumbered women by two to one. The ward catered for patients between 18 and 65 years of age, although many were aged between 20 and 35 years.

On entry to the ward, one was immediately aware of the high volume of noise and general hullabaloo, associated with many severely ill patients immersed in their own worlds, talking to imaginary people and occasionally appearing to act on what voices were telling them. Nurses seemed to spend much of their time running about trying to deal with distressed or aggressive patients in different parts of the ward. It seemed almost impossible to conduct therapeutic group sessions in the ward.

The pressure on beds was severe: the ward had the highest bed occupancy of any site – 153% – and one of the lowest average lengths of inpatient stay – 5.2 weeks (see Tables 4.3A–D). To deal with this level of demand, many patients slept in other wards, but it was more likely that they had been found beds in the private sector as extra contractual referrals, (ECRs). Some patients came into the ward during the day for treatment and their meals.

The ward cared for some of the most severely ill patients encountered at any site during the study (see Tables 4A–D): 62% had a dependency level of 2 or more, which meant that a majority of patients required some assistance with daily living activities, such as washing, eating and drinking; 54% were detained under a section of the 1983 Mental Health Act; 24% needed to be closely observed by staff because of the danger of self-harm or the potential danger posed to others; and 81% were diagnosed as suffering from schizophrenia. Staff reported that illicit drug use, drunkenness and incidents involving threatening behaviour with knives occurred in the ward. The field-work researchers were aware of at least three incidents involving patients being 'high' because of drink or drugs; each occasion required the intervention of two staff members.

The highly charged and difficult patient population took its toll on nursing staff; one reported that 'You can only stand this for two years or so, otherwise you'd burn out.' During fieldwork, the high propor-tion of unfilled permanent posts and the use of agency or bank nurses were notable features of a number of shifts. These circumstances were fairly typical of most inner-city study sites.

CASE STUDY 4.2

B6 was a ward in a traditional Water Tower hospital in a rural area; it also received admissions from a large city located some distance away. The ward cared for patients between 18 and 65 years of age, although many patients were over 40 years of age. There were slightly more men in the ward than women. It was rare for patients to be admitted from ethnic minority groups, and there were no patients from such groups in the ward.

On entering the ward, the calm and relaxed approach to nursing was in marked contrast to that of inner-city sites. Many patients attended therapeutic group activities organised by therapy staff in the hospital's occupational therapy department. Researchers often saw patients in the ward reviewing their programme of care with nursing staff.

Severe pressure on beds was rare, although the number of peaks in demand had increased in recent years: the ward had an 86% bed occupancy, close to the figure recommended by the Royal College of Psychiatrists, and also had a shorter average length of stay – 3.5 weeks (see Tables 4.3A–D). During their stay, most patients were able to recover fully prior to discharge so few were readmitted soon after leav-ing hospital.

The ward cared for the least severely ill patients of any study site (see Tables 4.4A–D): 54% had a dependency level of 2 or more, these being mainly older patients with physical ailments such as walking difficulties. Twenty-five per cent of the patients were detained, 12%

required close observation by ward staff, and 8% were diagnosed as schizophrenic. This less demanding patient population meant that nurses were more able to involve patients fully in all aspects of care. Nurses reported a greater satisfaction with the nursing role compared with their counterparts caring for more difficult populations. These circumstances were reasonably typical of sites located in rural settings.

One of the most significant differences between case studies 4.1 and 4.2 is in the nature of the work undertaken by staff. These comparisons, and indeed the whole study, confirm the many patient population changes and the impact of change on nurses' workloads reported in other studies (Hollander and Slater, 1994; Thornicroft and Strathdee, 1994; Johnson and Thornicroft, 1995; Powell et al., 1995; Lelliot et al., 1996). First, there has been increased pressure on beds owing to the reduction in the number of psychiatric beds, partly as a result of hospital closures. Second, as North et al. (1993), the Audit Commission (1994) and the Social Services Inspectorate (1995) indicated, the present study confirms that beds are increasingly blocked as a small proportion of patients remain unnecessarily in hospital because of the lack of suitable housing and other community services. Third, there has been a significant increase in the severity of illness of patients in wards, as confirmed by the Audit Commission (1994), Gournay (1994), Powell et al. (1995), Thomas et al. (1995), the Department of Health (1996a) and National Health Service Executive (1996). Finally, as a number of commentators have noted, there has been an increase in the number of detained patients in mental health wards (Barnes et al., 1990; Coid, 1993; Rogers et al., 1993; House of Commons Health Committee, 1994; Hopton, 1995; Mental Health Act Commission, 1995).

Perhaps unsurprisingly, staff who were caring for difficult populations in sites A1, B7, C9, C10 and C11 reported less satisfaction with their work. Job dissatisfaction had become increasingly associated with crisis intervention. This staff perception was borne out by fieldwork researchers who witnessed – or were aware of – numerous acts of crisis intervention undertaken by nurses. As pressure on beds intensified in recent years, stabilisation of patients' conditions prior to discharge, rather than nurses' involvement in the complete process of care, had become the norm.

Nurses with difficult populations also reported that the consequence of such developments was to squeeze the time available for nurse–patient contact, especially care planning (Audit Commission, 1994; Hollander and Slater, 1994; Lelliott et al. 1996). The volume of paperwork and additional administrative duties especially was identified as a problem (see Chapters 5 and 6). Thus the nurse–patient interaction that did occur was increasingly focused on discharge planning, with little time available for care planning or therapeutic conversation. Workload pressures were said to compromise the scope for patients' greater involvement in care planning, a finding consistent with those reported in other studies (Shields *et al.*, 1988; Higgins, 1993; Glenister, 1994; Higgins *et al.*, 1994; Jewell, 1994; Seed, 1994; Trnobranski, 1994; Hewison, 1995; Jarrett and Payne, 1995; Robinson, 1995). Nurses frequently referred to the dilemma between allowing patients sufficient time to recover before discharge, and discharging patients too early to release beds. This dilemma was identified as a severe problem at a number of sites, particularly in Region C. A nurse summed up this dilemma:

> The care team have to make some difficult judgements: is this patient well enough to cope outside, because we need the bed? It does lead to a revolving door syndrome in some cases. Some are discharged too early; community services can't cope; and they end up back on the ward in a few weeks.

Many nurses also spoke of the increasing dilemma encountered operating either a custodial or a therapeutic approach to care. Once again, this echoes the findings of recent studies (Shields *et al.*, 1988; Porter, 1993; Glenister, 1994; Jewell, 1994; Seed, 1994; Robinson, 1995). Nurses referred to the large number of detained patients currently in wards as evidence of the shift to a more custodial approach to care, even though detention was undertaken for sound clinical reasons (see Tables 4.3A–D; see also Mental Health Act Commission, 1995). Typical of the comments made by nurses on this subject was:

> We try to operate a therapeutic, patient-centred approach to care. But the current state of the ward often means that this seems to be compromised; many patients are detained – often for good reasons. It makes me feel uncomfortable of the way nursing is going. I didn't come into nursing to be like a prison warder. It certainly feels like that at times. I'm sure it contributes to the increasing level of violence and incidents in the ward by severely disturbed, detained patients.

The severe pressure on beds observed at many inner-city sites – A1, B7, C9, C10 and C11 – was not seen at most other sites. Staff caring for more manageable populations – A2, A3, A4, B6 and B8 – were generally able to maintain what they regarded as a more satisfying nursing role, one that involved them in the complete process of care, including spending time with patients in care planning and preparing them adequately for discharge in a therapeutic environment (see figures in Chapters 5 and 6). This staff perception was borne out by many observed instances of staff and patients discussing the latter's programme of care.

There was a noticeable difference between regions in terms of difficult and manageable patient populations. Thus, apart from A1, Region C sites cared for demonstrably more difficult populations compared with Region B sites, which cared for some of the most manageable populations (see Tables 4.3A–D and Tables 4.4A–D). As already mentioned in Chapter 3, Region C had witnessed the removal of many mental health beds. Even though staffing arrangements had been adjusted to deal with more severely ill patients, the sheer pressure on beds meant that staff were often unable adequately to undertake the complete process of care. Their overriding concern was to free beds to make way for more needy patients. (Chapters 5 and 6 deal more fully with staffing issues.) In contrast, Region B had one of the lowest reductions in bed numbers of any region, and also had one of the highest increases in the number of hospital nursing staff. Thus staff were more able to deal with the demands imposed on them and be involved in the complete process of care. (Tables 5.1A–C show the relatively high staff-to-patient ratio of Region B sites compared with sites in Regions A and C.)

Summary

- There were significant differences between the age, type and location of hospitals, shape and size of wards, and types of accommodation available to patients.
- Ward environments have an impact on patient recovery: Nightingale-type wards with communal sleeping areas were judged less satisfactory.
- There were observable differences between sites with difficult and those with manageable populations. The former were characterised by high bed occupancies, inner-city locations and severely ill patients. The latter had lower occupancies, suburban or rural locations and less severely ill patients.
- Region C, compared with Region B, had more severely ill patients. Changes in bed numbers and staffing levels within Regions B and C might account for the differences.
- The composition of the population had a profound impact on the nature of nurses' work. Staff at sites with difficult populations were

less involved in the complete process of care. Pressure on beds meant that their overriding consideration was freeing beds so that more needy patients could be admitted. Staff with manageable populations, on the other hand, were more involved in the complete process of care, and patients left the ward more fully recovered.

Chapter 5
Management and leadership

This chapter explores the following data to discuss the roles of senior ward nurses in acute mental health wards:

- interviews with ward staff;
- activity analysis;
- researchers' perceptions;
- staff questionnaires.

The responsibility for clinical management and leadership of nurses rested with senior, G and F grade, nurses. Their main tasks involved ensuring that the ward was appropriately staffed and the nurses adequately supported. These issues, and the perceived barriers to effective management and leadership, are discussed below.

Staff cover

Part of the senior nurses' role was matching available nursing resources to patients' needs. This included mainly bridging short-term gaps by using agency or bank staff and dealing with longer-term personnel issues such as the appointment of additional staff. G grade nurses were responsible for compiling duty rotas so that the ward had an appropriate staff mix for inpatient needs. G grade nurses considered this activity time-consuming because of the number of factors they had to take into account:

- the number, skills, grade and sex of staff and, at sites A1, C9, C10 and C11, staff who could speak a minority ethnic language;
- requests for specific days off or to work particular shifts;
- annual, study or maternity leave;
- staff on long-term sick leave and unforeseen short-term sickness;
- the needs of patients.

Senior ward nurses compiling the off duty rota was well established at most sites, but it had not been devolved to the G grade nurse at site A1, where it remained the responsibility of the H grade clinical nurse manager. The variety of staffing arrangements and the number and grades of staff on duty per shift – early, late and night – at each site during the week of fieldwork are shown in Tables 5.1A–C.

Table 5.1A Staff on early shift duty

Site	Mon	Tue	Wed	Thurs	Fri	Sat	Sun
A1	F	G	F		G	F	
	E	D	E	E D	D	D	E D
	A	A×2	A×2	A×2	A×2	A	A
A2	G	G	F	G F	G	F	F
	E×2	E	E D		E	E	E D
	A	A×2	A	A×2	A×2	A×2	A
A3	G	G			G		
	E×2 D	E D C	E D×2	E D×2	E	E×2 D	E×2
	A	A	C A×2	C A×2	A	A×2	C A×2
A4	G F	G	G F	G	G	F	F
	E×3	E×4	E×2 D	E×2 D	E×2 D	E×2 D	E×2 D
	A×2	B	A	B A	B A	A	A
B5	F	G F	F	G×2	G×2		
	E D	E D	E D	E	E×2	E×2	E
	B					B	B
B6	H		H	H	H		
	E D×2	E D	E D	E D	E D	E D	D×3
	A	A×2	A	A	A×2	A×2	A
B7	G F		G F	G	G F		
	E	E D		E	E	E	E D
	A	A	A×2	A	A	A×2	A
B8		G	F	G	G	F	
	E×3	E×2 D	E×3 D	E D	E×2	E×2 D	E×2
	A×2	A×2	A	A	A×3	A	A
C9	G	G F	F	F	G F	G	G
	E×3	E D×2	E×2 D	E×2 D	E D	E×2 D	E D
							A

(contd)

Table 5.1A (contd)

Site	Mon	Tue	Wed	Thurs	Fri	Sat	Sun
C10	G	F	G F	G F	G F		
	E×3	D	E×2	E	E D	E×2 D	E×2
	A	A×2		A	A		A
C11	G F	G	G	G	G	F	F
	E D	E×2 D	E D×2	D×3	D×4	D×3	D×3
	C						

Key: 1. Grades per shift are indicated by the relevant letter H to A. 2. Number per shift is obtained by counting the letters in each box, for example: Table 5.1A, site A1, Monday, staff on duty: F, E and A = 3. 3. A letter and number together, for example: E×2, shows that two E grade nurses were on duty.

A1: G grade nurse worked 09.00–17.00 hrs, Monday–Friday; F grade nurse worked only day shifts; internal rotation had recently been introduced; permanent night staff were employed.

A2: G/F grade nurses worked only day shifts, internal rotation was well established; no permanent night staff were employed.

A3: G/F grade nurses worked only day shifts, internal rotation had recently been introduced; no permanent night staff were employed. The ward had additional responsibilities to provide staff cover for the ECT suite, and for a two-bed mother and baby unit (there were no admissions during fieldwork).

A4: G grade nurse worked 08.00–16.00 hrs, Monday–Friday; internal rotation was well established; permanent night staff were employed. The ward had an additional responsibility to provide staff cover for the ECT suite.

B5: All staff worked either permanent days or permanent nights.

B6: H grade nurse worked 09.00–17.00 hrs, Monday–Friday and was also clinical team leader for two other acute ward; internal rotation was well established; no permanent night staff were employed.

B7: G grade nurse worked 09.00–17.00 hrs, Monday–Friday; all other staff worked either permanent days or permanent nights.

B8: G/F grade nurses worked only day shifts; internal rotation was well established; no permanent night staff were employed.

C9: G/F grade nurse worked only day shifts and also acted as duty nurse for emergency admissions to the unit; internal rotation was well established; no permanent night staff were employed.

C10: G grade nurse worked 09.00–17.00 hrs, Monday–Friday and G/F grade nurses also acted as duty nurses for emergency admissions to the unit; internal rotation was well established; no permanent night staff were employed.

C11: G grade nurse worked 09.00–17.00 hrs, Monday–Friday and also acted as senior nurse site manager for 1 or 2 days per week; internal rotation had recently been introduced; no permanent night staff were employed.

Table 5.1B Staff on late shift duty

Site	Mon	Tue	Wed	Thurs	Fri	Sat	Sun
A1	G D A×2	F E A×2	E D A×2	G D A×2	E D A	E D A	F D A
A2	F D A×2	G D A×2	F E A×2	E×2 D A	F E A×2	G E A×2	E×2 D A
A3	G E×2 D×2 A	G E×2 A	E D×2 C A	E×2 D×2 A	G E D×2 C A	E×2 D A×2	E×2 C A×2
A4	F E D B A	F E D A	E×2 B A	E D×2 A	E×2 D A	E×3 D A	E×2 D A×2
B5	E D A	G E	G E	G E	E B	F B	G A
B6	E D A×2	E D A×2	E D A×2	E D A×2	E D×2 A	E D×2 A	F E D A
B7	E D A	F D A	E A	F A×2	E D A	E A	E D A
B8	G D A×2	F E D A×2	G E D A×2	F E×2 A	F E D A×2	E×3 D A×2	E×2 D A
C9	F E×3 D	F E×2	E×2 D×2	G F E D	F E D×2	E×3 D	E×2 D A
C10	F E×2 A	G E×2	E×3 A×2	E×2 A	E×2 A	E×2 A	E×2 A
C11	E×2 D A	E D×2	E×2 D	F E D A	F D A	E D×2 A	E D×3 A

See Table 5.1A for explanation.

Table 5.1C Staff on night shift duty

Site	Mon	Tue	Wed	Thurs	Fri	Sat	Sun
A1							
	E	E	E	E	E	E	E
	A×2	A×2	A×2	A×2	A×2	A×2	A×2
A2							
	E	E	E	E	E	E	E
	A×2	A×2	A×2	A×2	A×2	A×2	A×2
A3							
	E	E	E	E	E	E	E
	A	A	A	A	A	A	A
A4	F	F	F	F	F	F	F
	D	D	D	D	D	D	D
	A	A	A	A	A	A	A
B5							
	E	E	E	E	E	E	E
	A	A	A	A	A	A	A
B6							
	E	E	E	D	D	E	E
	A×2	A×2	A×2	A×2	A×2	A×2	A×2
B7							
	E	E	E	E	E	E	E
	A	A	A	A	A	A	A
B8							
	E	E	E	E	E	E	E
	A×2	A×2	A×2	A×2	A×2	A×2	A×2
C9							
	E×2	E×2 D	E×2 D	E D	E×2 D	E×2 D	E×2 D
C10							
	E	D	E	E	E	E	E
	A	A	A	A	A	A	A
C11							
	E×2 D C	E×2 D	E D	E D	E D	E D	E×3 D
	C				C	C	

Tables 5.1A–C demonstrate a number of interesting points

1. G and F grade nurses mostly worked day shifts.
2. A number of senior nurses had additional duties. The H grade nurse at B6 was also clinical team leader for two other acute wards, G and F grade nurses at C9 and C10 acted as duty nurses for emergency admissions, and the G grade nurse at C11 acted as senior nurse site manager for 1 or 2 days per week, which involved being on call and dealing with all the nursing problems in the hospital.
3. Internal rotation was the principal means of organising staff cover (except for sites B5 and B7). This method was well established at A2, A4, B6, B8, C9 and C10. It had only recently been introduced at A1, A3 and C11, but permanent night staff were still employed at A1, A4 and C11.
4. Early and late shifts were the busiest, especially if a MDT meeting (ward round) was scheduled, which usually lasted for the whole morning or afternoon. Additional staff were usually on duty at these times because at least one member of staff – usually a G, F or E grade nurse – was involved in the meeting. Weekends and night shifts were usually quiet and therefore fewer staff were on duty.
5. The lack of unqualified staff on duty was a notable feature of Region C: the complex and demanding needs of patients called for the skills and expertise of experienced nurses. A1, which also cared for a demanding patient population, had not made these kinds of adjustment. Most other sites often had two unqualified staff on duty during day shifts despite the fact that staff at most inner-city sites, especially A1, C9, C10 and C11, were dealing with difficult patients (see Tables 4.3A–D and 4.4A–D). Here, staff seemed under particular pressure dealing with a large number of severely ill patients.
6. Staff at A3 and A4 had additional responsibilities providing staff cover for the ECT suite, and A3 provided staff cover for a two-bed mother and baby unit.
7. There were many agency and bank staff on duty in Region C. Problems of staff recruitment and retention, and the extent of labour market competition within the capital were cited as the reasons.

Organisational arrangements

A primary nursing arrangement was in operation in all the sites. In accordance with a key standard contained in the Patient's Charter (Department of Health, 1992c), every patient on admission was allocated to a named, primary nurse, although the term 'key worker' was also used in some sites. The definition of primary nursing closest to that described by nurses was that of Marriner-Tomey (1988, pp. 149–50):

Primary nursing features a registered nurse who gives total patient care to four to six patients while she is on duty. She remains responsible for the care of those patients 24 hours a day throughout the patient's hospitalization. The associate nurse cares for the patient by using the care plan developed by the primary nurse while the primary nurse is off duty. The associate nurse is to contact the primary nurse regarding changes in the care plan.

Interestingly, nursing assistants acted as associate workers at some sites (see Chapter 6 for a discussion of the role of the nursing assistant).

The focus of the named nurse, clear to nurses themselves, was the plan of care for individual patients. Named nurses:

- devised the care plan;
- monitored progress;
- evaluated regularly the goals negotiated with the patient (see Chapter 6 for a full discussion of the role of the named nurse).

The involvement of the patient was encouraged throughout (Department of Health, 1994a). The named nurse was charged with feeding back information concerning a patient's progress to other members of the multidisciplinary care team at its weekly meeting or ward round. Ward staff also belonged to a nursing team that related to a particular consultant.

Some commentators report confusion concerning primary nursing definitions. Thomas and Bond (1990), for example, found that operational definitions of primary nursing were lacking when they carried out their study on the organisation of nursing care and the organisation of staffing in hospital wards. They identified six criteria that help to distinguish task allocation, team nursing and primary nursing:

1. grouping nurses and deciding the length of allocation to specific patients;
2. allocating nursing work;
3. organising the duty rota;
4. nursing accountability for patient care;
5. updating patients' care plans;
6. liaison with medical and other staff.

Thomas and Bond (1990, p. 1110) concluded that:

In order to provide replicable research into the organisation of nursing care, it is essential to identify whether discrete types actually exist and to define what operational features are characteristic of each organisational method ... results show that the organisation of nursing in few wards fulfils five or more of the criteria for inclusion in a particular modality.

Thomas and Bond urged caution when drawing conclusions from studies about the organisation of nursing care unless the type of nursing care was clearly defined and adequately described.

Echoing the findings of other studies, senior nurses in the present study identified a number of practical difficulties with primary nursing in acute psychiatric wards:

* arranging duty rotas so that a primary or associate nurse was on duty;
* enabling all primary nurses to attend MDT meetings;
* the effect of staff sickness, annual leave and maternity leave on maintaining primary nursing;
* sharing information with all those involved with each patient;
* the emphasis on multidisciplinary working meaning that it was difficult to assign blame to one nurse if primary nursing did not operate optimally.

In the light of these difficulties, if neither the primary nurse nor the associate worker was available for a particular patient, the patient was assigned to any available nurse. The following comment by a named nurse was typical:

> While we operate and call it primary nursing, it's really a kind of hybrid primary nursing. You have someone who is the named nurse, the primary nurse, but because we work in teams, we can step in to work with most patients, if required. At the end of the day patients often only want someone to talk to. They don't differentiate between nurses. It is only with respect to care planning that primary nursing becomes important.

Service development

Senior nurses were responsible for developing and implementing nursing and related policies issues, and for ensuring that staff that had the requisite skills to carry them out. Examples of such policies were:

* reviewing criteria for which patients should be placed on high levels of observation, as this involved high-cost, one-to-one nursing cover;
* developing a team structure, which (a) corresponded with consultants' geographical catchment areas, and (b) responded to legislative requirements;
* the CPA.

Owing to the demanding nature of the patient population at some sites (see Chapter 4), and the volume of paperwork that all senior nurses were required to complete (see below), it was often difficult for senior ward nurses to adopt a proactive, planned approach to service development. Instead, a reactive, crisis management approach was the norm. The following comment was typical of those made by senior nurses:

> In recent times – because of the client mix and staffing levels – it's staff support and service development that tends to slip. You adopt a 'we'll deal with issues as they arise' style. A more systematic approach to service development, in terms of making sure that staff and patients are appropriately matched, has become more difficult as these become increasingly out of synch with provided funding. I feel at times that I'm a juggler: trying to juggle the available resources so that a reasonably safe therapeutic environment is provided for patients. That's my hope anyway.

Staff support

A number of pressures took a toll on staff:

- the difficult patient populations (see Chapter 4);
- peaks in demand resulting from increasing, unplanned, emergency admissions;
- the volume of paperwork that staff were required to complete (see below and also Chapter 6).

Such pressures resulted in unexpected staff sickness and meant that adjustments to staffing were required at short notice. All senior nurses had to contend with workforce planning difficulties and arrange extra staff cover. One grade G nurse said that:

> The changing patient population and unforeseen peaks in demand make it difficult to provide a decent environment for patients and staff. I think maintaining, or at least trying to keep the ward in order, is necessary for patient recovery. It means that you need to keep a close eye on what's happening. It's not easy to do when the ward is busy.

The pressures imposed on ward staff raised the issue of what support and supervision were available to them. Although no data about staff sickness were available from sites, a worrying trend identified by senior nurses was the increase in stress and staff sickness arising from the unpredictability of the working environment.

Stress and staff sickness

The nature and effect of organisational change on staff within the public sector in general, and the health service in particular, has been the focus of a number of recent studies (Handy, 1991; Audit Commission, 1994; House of Commons Health Committee, 1994; Kirby and Pollock, 1995; Leary *et al.*, 1995; Fowler, 1996; Orton 1996). For nurses, the turmoil associated with the rapid change emanating from the 1991 health service reforms was seen as a significant contributory factor in the increasing pressures. The health service reforms had increased pressures on staff in the following ways:

- those pressures resulting from organisational restructuring, for example the move to Trust status for many hospitals and the devolution of responsibilities to ward level (see below);
- those owing to the introduction of new working practices that resulted in extra administrative responsibilities for staff, such as the system of named nurses and the CPA (see Chapter 6);
- those resulting from the changing expectations of service users with respect to health service workers, for example the new rights and complaints procedures introduced by the Patient's Charter (Department of Health, 1992c; see also Chapter 6).

Although a number of studies noted the association of organisational turbulence with increased stress and stress-related illnesses among health service workers, including nurses (Handy, 1991; Kirby and Pollock, 1995; Leary *et al.*, 1995; Fowler, 1996; Orton, 1996), few examined the effects of such change on hospital mental health nurses (Leary *et al.*, 1995).

In the current study, many nurses admitted that they had taken occasional days sick leave during the previous year. Owing to the demanding nature of their current workload, recourse to such coping strategies was necessary but taken with great reluctance. Orton (1996) noted that such a coping strategy, to relieve pressure, was commonly employed by workers in many industrial settings. The following was typical of the comments expressed by nurses:

> At times you feel burned out. Your batteries need recharging, so you take a day or two off sick. I don't like doing this because you are adding to the problems of colleagues and friends, who may also feel the same. Without the time out you are liable to crack under the pressure.

A number of senior ward staff were monitoring staff sickness more systematically and had noticed a trend. When particularly difficult patients were admitted, they noticed a rise in the level of short-term sickness. Rix's (1987) study of violent incidents in a regional secure unit found that short-term staff sickness levels rose sharply as more demanding patients were admitted. More worryingly, the high turnover of staff in Region C, referred to above, was being linked to the same phenomenon. Senior nurses were rarely critical of other staff for resorting to such measures. As one remarked:

> You can only put up with this for so long: 2 or 3 years at the most – then you need a change. What we have to deal with in the ward does take it out of you both physically and mentally. I know after I've done a week or two of this you need a break. Staff all have their ways of coping with it: going for a drink, time off sick, whatever.

Informants confessed to being at a loss to know what to do about this problem. Offering support to colleagues and making sure that staff felt equipped to deal with the pressures were, however, used.

Clinical supervision

F grade nurses both led and clinically supervised staff. Specifically, G grade nurses provided clinical supervision for F grade nurses, and the H grade clinical nurse manager supervised G grade nurses. A system of individual performance review (IPR) operated in all sites (Department of Health, 1994a; Mental Health Foundation, 1994; Darley, 1995; Northcott, 1996; United Kingdom Central Council for Nursing, Midwifery and Health Visiting, 1996). IPR involved an examination, usually at monthly intervals, of the staff's clinical work and developmental needs.

Owing to pressures on their time, many senior nurses had difficulty finding sufficient time to undertake staff supervision (see below). This meant that clinical supervision occurred less frequently than they wished. At times, supervision consisted of supporting staff on a day-to-day basis in an *ad hoc* way, especially helping staff who had been involved in serious untoward incidents such as being hit by a patient. Fortunately, however, to protect themselves against attacks from unpredictable patients, many nurses had been educated in control and restraint (C and R) techniques; otherwise the situations might have been worse.

Hospital staff in Region A were unsure about what counselling support, if any, was available to them, other than that offered by ward colleagues. In Regions B and C, staff counsellors – usually psychologists – were available for those who required support. However, peer support by ward colleagues remained the principal means of support at all sites.

Barriers to effective management and leadership

Other studies have shown that ward management was reported by senior nurses to be in a state of flux, reflecting the more general condition of nursing (Mangan, 1993; Palmer, 1993; Roberts, 1993; Stewart, 1993). The introduction of Griffiths-style general management, and the move to flatter management structures from the mid-1980s (Griffiths, 1983), paved the way for responsibilities and decision-making to be increasingly devolved to ward level.

A number of studies (Jones 1990; Audit Commission, 1991; Roberts, 1993; Department of Health, 1996b) also suggested that the drive to reduce public sector organisations' overheads, particularly management and other administrative costs, had had an impact on the NHS. Senior nurses in the present study reported that resource centres had been created within their hospitals. Resource centres consisted of individual wards' or groups of wards' financial information. Managers of resource centres were responsible for operational aspects, including personnel and finance, that had previously been handled centrally. Thus devolution of responsibilities to ward level had a significant impact on the role of senior ward nurses. Their managerial and administrative duties increasingly conflicted with their role as senior clinicians, particularly in terms of service development and clinical supervision (see above). Senior informants questioned whether the delayering NHS management structures had gone too far. The issue of additional paperwork and administrative duties was a major, related issue for E and D grade nurses (see Chapter 6).

The pressure for senior nurses to adopt an administrative rather than a clinical role was overwhelming. The question of whether ward managers (G grade nurses) needed to be nurses was raised during the interviews (see also Audit Commission, 1991). G grade nurse informants stressed that qualified nurses both managed and led ward staff. Also, they helped other staff when the ward was busy. It was important, therefore, for senior nurses to:

- maintain their nursing knowledge and skills;
- develop ward services;
- offer advice;

- support and train other staff;
- assess the implications of developments.

Senior staff were concerned that their managerial and administrative duties might eventually squeeze the time available for their role as clinical leaders and their involvement in direct, hands-on patient care.

Figures 5.1 and 5.2 illustrate the decrease in the amount of time that G and F grade nurses respectively spent in direct patient care over the period 1985–96:

- 1985–89: 29% and 44.9%;
- 1990–93: 17.3% and 34.4%;
- 1994–96: 5.7% and 22.6%.

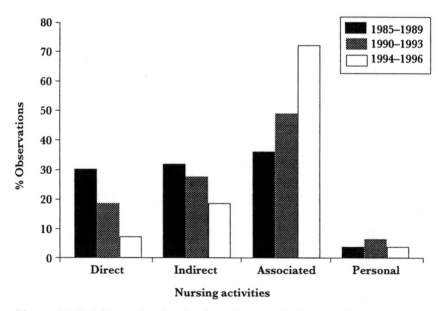

Figure 5.1 Activities undertaken by G grade nurses during recorded observations, 1985–96

Notes:
1. Categories used in Figures 5.1–5.10 and 6.1–6.20.
D: *Direct patient care: one-to-one contact between staff and patient*: one-to-one discussions between staff and patient, care planning, assessment, comforting/controlling patient, crisis intervention; group sessions in ward; dispensing medication to patients; observations of patients; assistance with patients' personal care; escorting patient off ward for treatment; staff recreation with a patient or group of patients; ECT.
I: *Indirect patient care: discussions between staff about patients*: ward round; shift hand-overs; discussion between staff and relatives about a patient.
A: *Associated work: work that is not directly related to patient care, but is nevertheless important for the delivery of nursing care*: meetings with medical staff or other professionals, or between

(contd)

ward staff; office duties; teaching student nurses; domestic duties; off ward: duty
nurse (Region C only); errands.
P: *Personal time*; staff breaks.
2. Obs = percentage of recorded observations.
3. Data sources: *All activities*: 1985–93, Hurst (1995a); 1994–96, present study. *Regions*:
A, Yorkshire; B, Northern; C, London. *Geographical location of hospital*: IC, Inner city:
A1, B7, C9, C10 and C11; OU, Other urban: A4 and B5; R, Rural: A2, A3, B6 and
B8. *Hospital type*: DGH, District general hospital: A2, B7, B8 and C9; WT, Water
Tower: A3, B6 and C11; O, Other hospital settings: A1, A4, B5 and C10. *Bed occupan-
cies*: = 100%: A1, B5, C9, C10 and C11; < 100%: A2, A3, A4, B6, B7 and B8.

In Appendix 15, Hurst (1995a) gives data for the years 1985–93,
including a detailed breakdown of the four categories used in the
figures in Chapters 5 and 6: direct patient care, indirect patient care,
associated work and personal time.

Figures 5.3–5.10 below show the time that G and F grade nurses
spent in activities such as direct patient care during the period 1994–96.
These data are explained by region, geographical location of hospital,
hospital type and bed occupancy (see also Appendix 15). They reveal
some interesting patterns among direct patient care activities.

Region

- Overall, G grade nurses spent little time in direct patient care
  (Figure 5.3), the figure in Region B being highest: 13.5% compared
  with 4.8% and 7.5% respectively for Regions A and C.

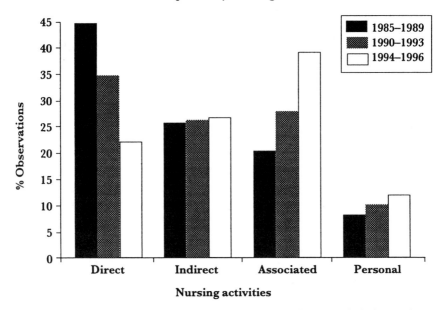

Figure 5.2 Activities undertaken by F grade nurses during recorded observations,
1985–96

- Grade F nurses in Regions B and C in particular (Figure 5.4) spent the most time in direct patient care: 35.5% and 29.3% respectively.

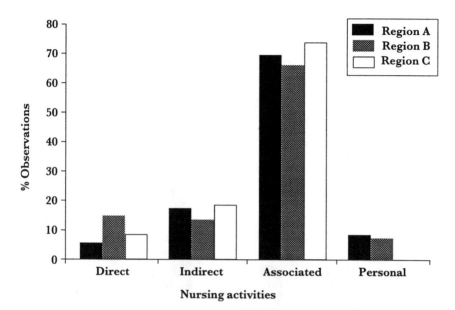

Figure 5.3 Activities undertaken by G grade nurses during recorded observations by Region, 1994–96

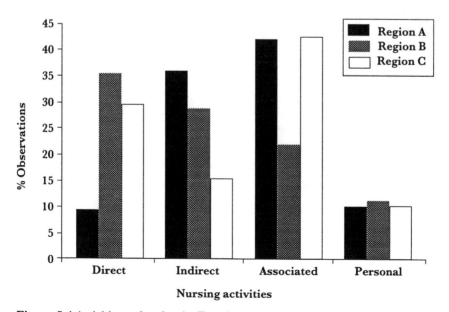

Figure 5.4 Activities undertaken by F grade nurses during recorded observations by region, 1994–96

Geographical location of hospital

- Grade G nurses in inner-city sites (Figure 5.5), spent the least time in direct patient care: 5.7% compared with the respective figures for other urban and rural sites – 17.2% and 6.5%.
- Grade F nurses in inner-city sites (Figure 5.6) spent the most time in direct patient care activities: 29.3% compared with the corresponding figures for other urban and rural sites of 35.5% and 9.4%.

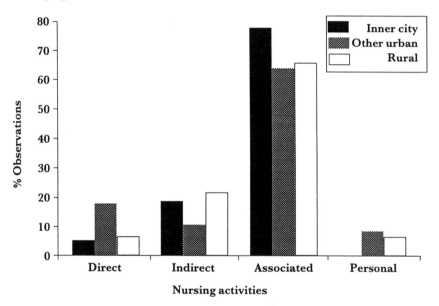

Figure 5.5 Activities undertaken by G grade nurses during recorded observations by geographical location of hospital, 1994–96

Hospital type

- Grade G nurses in district general hospital sites (Figure 5.7) spent the most time in direct patient care: 13.5% compared with sites located in Water Tower hospitals and other service settings – 6.0% and 9.7% respectively.
- Grade F nurses in other service settings (Figure 5.8) spent the most time undertaking direct patient care activities: 26.1% compared with the figure for those located in district general hospitals – 17.3%. (There were no F grade nurses on duty during the fieldwork undertaken in Water Tower hospitals.)

Bed occupancies

- Grade G nurses at sites with an occupancy of 100% or more (Figure 5.9) – A1, B5, C9, C10 and C11 – spent more time carrying out direct patient care: 8.7% compared with sites with an occupancy below 100%, for which the figure was 6.5%.

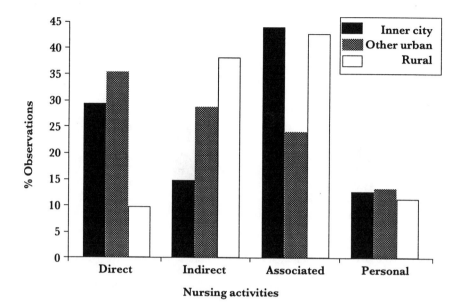

Figure 5.6 Activities undertaken by F grade nurses during recorded observations by geographical location of hospital, 1994–96

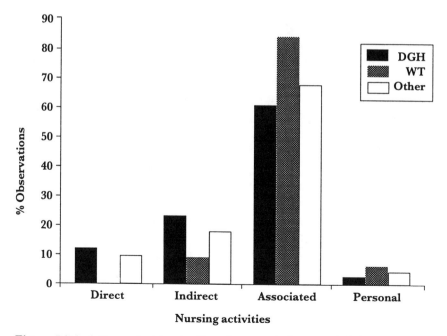

Figure 5.7 Activities undertaken by G grade nurses during recorded observations by hospital type, 1994–96

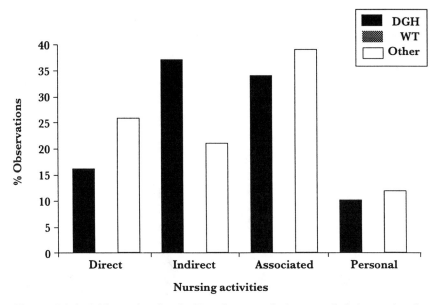

Figure 5.8 Activities undertaken by F grade nurses during recorded observations by hospital type, 1994–96

- Grade F nurses at sites with an occupancy of 100% or more spent over three times the amount of time in direct patient care (Figure 5.10): 31.1% compared with their counterparts at sites with an occupancy below 100% – 9.4%.

Figures 5.3–5.10 show that F grade nurses spent the most time in direct patient care compared with their G grade colleagues. This was perhaps related to their assigned clinical leader roles. The graphs also highlight a reasonably strong relationship between G grade nurses working in inner-city, district general hospitals with a bed occupancy of over 100% and spending more time undertaking direct patient care activities, compared with the situation in other settings. The greater pressure on other ward staff was perhaps significant. Grade G nurses in Region C also devoted more time to direct patient care compared with those in Regions A and B. Again, this perhaps reflected the greater pressures on other ward staff in Region C. (A discussion of the volume of paperwork undertaken by G and F grade nurses is provided below.) However, the same relationships were much stronger for F grade nurses. The greater pressures on other staff might explain this situation, but the clinical leader role might also have been an important factor.

Two aspects of devolution had a significant impact on the clinical leadership and direct patient care duties of G and F grade nurses. First was their increased responsibility, accountability and authority for what happened in the wards. Second was the volume of paperwork and additional administrative duties they undertook.

Responsibility, accountability and authority

Devolution of responsibilities had both positive and negative effects on ward management. The greater freedom that senior nurses had to develop ward services, for example compiling staff duty rotas, employing additional staff and, at some sites, managing the ward budget, were

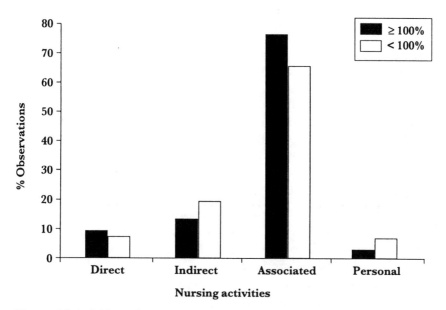

Figure 5.9 Activities undertaken by G grade nurses during recorded observations by bed occupancy level, 1994–96

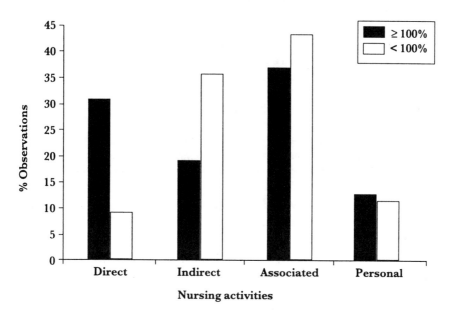

Figure 5.10 Activities undertaken by F grade nurses during recorded observations by bed occupancy level, 1994–96

welcomed. In contrast, their increasing administrative duties were vehemently disliked (see below), confirming what previous nursing studies (Roberts, 1993; Stewart, 1993; Hydes, 1995) had found. One G grade nurse summed up her colleagues' views:

> The extra responsibilities for the ward – staff planning, ward policies, budget management, etc. – have positives and negatives. It's good because I have more autonomy to develop ward services. However, a lot of the paperwork I have is often fairly mundane and much of the information has to be provided for various managers, but in different forms. I often feel that I could spend my time more effectively instead of engaged in a paper chase.

Views expressed by those who had increased responsibilities and the authority to act without first recourse to others – one site in Region A (A4), three sites in Region B (B5, B6 and B7) and all sites in Region C – were different from those of the nurses who lacked the authority to act independently: three sites in Region A (A1, A2 and A3) and one in Region B (B8). Duff (1995, pp. 49–50) addressed the relationship between responsibility, accountability and authority. Using the work of Lewis and Batey (1982a, 1982b) as her starting point, she argued that increased responsibilities also entail greater accountability. The mark of evolving professionalism, however, was the extent to which nurses had the authority to make decisions without first seeking the approval of their superiors or peers, for example medical staff and senior managers. The issue raised by Duff, therefore, is the difference between nurses recounting an event or decision and accounting for it. The former:

> is initiated by others; it carries the implication of error, and it occurs when people are called to task and asked to recreate and justify their actions, plans and goals.

Accounting for decisions, in contrast:

> implies that the person making the disclosure has both authority and autonomy in the areas of responsibility. To be accountable denotes an acceptance of the obligation to disclose and of the possible consequences of disclosure.

Having the autonomy to exercise discretion was closely related to the pace and nature of devolution. The pace varied noticeably across sites and had a regional pattern. In Region A especially, senior nurses often had the responsibility, but their ability to act autonomously was limited. This was in marked contrast to the situation in Region C and, to a lesser degree, Region B, where direct control over the ward budget meant having the responsibility and authority to act independently.

In Regions B and C, most G grade nurses had direct control over all aspects of staff and financial planning, including compiling duty rotas and meeting shortfalls in staffing, either temporarily (by the use of bank and agency staff) or permanently (by recruiting additional nurses). No G grade nurse in Region A had control over the ward budget. However, the G grade nurse at A4 was soon to acquire control, and, as already noted, at one site in Region A the G grade nurse did not have the authority to compile shift rotas, although he was soon to take on this responsibility. However, informants pointed out that they influenced staff recruitment decisions through their presence on interview panels.

The Audit Commission (1991) also identified the problem of how the incomplete devolution of responsibilities to ward managers can affect their ability to make the best use of ward resources if they lack authority for all aspects of staffing and finances. The issue of devolving ward budgets to G grade nurses was seen by the Commission to link responsibility and authority.

Grade G nurses also spoke of the link between the increased devolution of responsibilities for the ward to them and their greater accountability and authority for what happened in the ward (Bergman, 1981; Evans, 1993). They emphasised that their increased responsibilities for the ward had changed their relationship with other professionals, particularly medical staff. Decision-making had shifted from being predominantly medically led to the situation in which nursing inputs were increasingly important or, at the very least, the notion of shared accountability was emphasised. The move to multidisciplinary working was a significant development (see Chapter 6), as has been noted in other nursing studies (Read, 1995; Reed, 1995; Samson, 1995).

In Region C in particular, and inner-city sites in general – where bed occupancies were high and pressure on beds severe – senior nurses were more willing to challenge the decisions of medical staff (especially those relating to ward admissions) than were those at other sites, where the pressure on beds was not as acute. The grounds for questioning medical decisions were the risks to and the safety of staff and patients in the ward. On five occasions during fieldwork in Region C, researchers observed senior nurses challenging medical staff about potential admissions on safety grounds. Eventually, the medical staff accepted that there was a danger to staff and patients, and agreed to seek alternative locations for the admission. This was a difficult task because most sites already had bed occupancies in excess of 100% (see Tables 4.3A–D). The senior nurses' increasing gate-keeping role with respect to admission is discussed further in Chapter 6.

Rodgers (1995) noted that whenever a group of workers is subject to significant organisational change, issues of what training, skills and expertise are necessary to fulfil the new role inevitably arise (see Table 6.1 for the qualifications obtained by nursing staff, including those of senior nurses; see also Chapter 6). Notwithstanding the dilemma senior nurses expressed concerning the balance between their clinical and administrative roles, many of them in Regions B and C had obtained managerial qualifications. Few, on the other hand, had received specific training or adequate support from their employers to prepare them for their management role. Not only was the acquisition of such qualifications considered important in their work, but so was an acknowledgement of the direction in which their role was heading. This was not to say, however, that senior nurses wholeheartedly viewed their large managerial workload as a positive development. The overwhelming sense of administrative duties being a 'burden and getting in the way of why I came into nursing' was a sentiment frequently expressed. As a result, the greater autonomy senior nurses had for ward services was perceived negatively because of its association with increased paperwork, a finding consistent with that recorded in previous nursing studies (Jones, 1990; Roberts, 1993).

Paperwork and administrative duties

The findings confirm those of previous studies that senior nurses identify a strong link between their greater responsibilities for the ward and the increase in their administrative duties (Pickering and Fox, 1987; Audit Commission, 1991; Hurst, 1993a; Watson, 1995). Figures 5.1 and 5.2 above illustrate the rising levels of associated work, particularly office duties, for G and F grade nurses respectively over the period 1985–96:

- 1985–89: 33.3% and 22%;
- 1990–93: 47.7% and 28.4%;
- 1994–96: 72.3% and 37.3%.

Figures 5.3–5.10 above highlight the following variations among G and F grade nurses' work by region, by geographical location of hospital, by hospital type and by bed occupancy.

Region

- There were no significant regional variations for G grade nurses (see Figure 5.3 above). Approximately 70% of their time was devoted to associated work, including office duties.

- Grade F nurses in Region A had the most (43%) and Region C the least (11%) time devoted to office duties (see Figure 5.4 above).

Geographical location of hospital

- If off-ward duties were excluded, G and F grade nurses in inner-city sites spent the least time on associated work (see Figure 5.5 above) – 57.4% and 15% respectively – compared with their counterparts in other urban locations (64.3% and 22.6%) and rural areas (66.3% and 43%).

Hospital type

- Grade G nurses in district general hospital sites spent the least time undertaking associated work activities (see Figure 5.7 above) – 60.9% – compared with those in Water Tower hospitals (84.5%) and other service settings (67.4%).
- If off-ward activities were excluded, F grade nurses in other service settings spent the least time carrying out associated work duties (see Figure 5.8 above): 20.7% compared with 34.2% for those in district general hospital sites. (There were no F grade nurses on duty during fieldwork at the Water Tower hospitals.)

Bed occupancies

- Grade G nurses at sites with bed occupancies at or above 100% spent the most time undertaking associated work activities (see Figure 5.9 above) – 75.6% – compared with the figure for their counterparts at sites with a below 100% occupancy level, of 65.5%.
- If off-ward duties were excluded, F grade nurses at sites with bed occupancies at or above 100% spent the least time undertaking associated work activities (see Figure 5.10 above): 17.9% compared with those at sites with below 100% occupancy level – 43%.

Figures 5.3–5.10 show that F grade nurses spent the least time carrying out associated work activities, irrespective of region, type or location of hospital and bed occupancy, compared with their G grade nurse colleagues. The role of F grade nurses as clinical leaders was perhaps significant. The figures also highlight a reasonably strong relationship between G and F grade nurses working in inner-city, district general hospitals with bed occupancies in excess of 100% and devoting more time to associated work duties. The greater pressures on other staff were perhaps significant. In other words, the busier the site, the less paperwork and other administrative activities G and F grade nurses were able to complete.

The difficulty in balancing senior clinical ward manager roles was a concern to all G and F grade nurses, a finding consistent with other nursing studies (Wainwright *et al.*, 1986; Jones, 1990; Palmer, 1993; Roberts, 1993; Hydes, 1995). Indeed, Roberts (1993, p. 30) argued that the role of G grade nurses has increasingly become that of a 'middle manager and administrator' with operational responsibilities, and that this development has been reinforced by referring to G grade nurses as 'ward managers'. At all but one site – A1 – the G grade nurse was known as ward manager.

All G grade nurses expressed concern that their clinical role was taking second place to their managerial and administrative duties (see Figures 5.1, 5.3, 5.5, 5.7 and 5.9 above). At only two sites were G grade staff named nurses: A2 and B5. Hydes (1995) also noted the conflict that many G grade nurses encountered between their managerial and administrative and clinical roles (see also Hurst, 1995c). Managerial duties often required them to spend time away from the ward attending meetings with other G grade nurses and senior managers to discuss service developments. Figure 5.1 above illustrates the increasing time spent attending meetings for G grade nurses:

- 1985–89: 4.7%;
- 1990–93: 8.8%;
- 1994–96: 17%.

However, the clinical role of both G and F grade nurses – particularly in Region C – had been extended. They acted as the on-call nurse for emergency admissions into their respective units (Figures 5.3 and 5.4; see also Chapter 6).

Providing written records was acknowledged by senior nurses to be a requirement of an accountable profession, open to both internal and external scrutiny for purposes of quality assurance (see also Kitson, 1986; Pearson, 1987; Mead, 1990; Naylor *et al.*, 1991). According to Chalmers (1995, p. 35), the confidence exposed to external scrutiny was a measure of 'professional maturity'. Nevertheless, all G and F grade nurses said that many of their administrative duties were burdensome and that between 50% and 66% of their paperwork was not directly relevant to patient care. Indeed, a recent government report (Department of Health, 1996b) drew attention to the unnecessary bureaucracy that burdened the NHS. This was an aspect of senior nurses' work with which nurses were least satisfied. Such paperwork was often routine and completed for the benefit of others, for example senior managers in the hospital's finance and personnel departments. As a result of attending the feedback session for fieldwork sites in Regions A and B, one Trust Chief Executive of a participating site went into the acute wards of his local hospital the next day and decided that much of the paperwork completed by senior nurses was inappropriate. He planned to provide ward clerks to undertake such routine administrative duties.

Senior nurses questioned whether form-filling was an effective use of their time. They were particularly concerned because these activities took them away from patient contact and from providing clinical leadership to nursing staff. These issues exacerbated pressures on other staff (see Figures 5.1–5.10 above). The following two comments were typical:

> The amount of paperwork that I'm now required to do has increased a lot over the last few years. At one level, I don't mind that, it's important to be accountable for what you do. But on another level, much of it is unrelated to patient care, it's about providing feedback on service use to managers: the bed status, admissions and discharges, number of patients detained, use of bank and agency staff and so on.
>
> I think the [health service] reforms and the move to Trust status is largely responsible for the increase in paperwork. The business and financial culture means that managers are more cost conscious and concerned with providing value for money and this means that we must justify – in writing – how resources are used. My own view is that at times these considerations drive the system rather than concern for providing quality care for patients.

The issue of defensive practice mentioned above was also highlighted by other ward staff with respect to patient care (see Chapter 6).

While the volume of paperwork was of concern, of even greater concern was duplication. Senior nurses expressed frustration about requests for similar information, presented in slightly different ways, from different managers. Managers often expected such information to be provided on a shift or daily basis, including that on

- bed status: numbers of admissions and discharges;
- the use of bank and agency staff;
- the number of detained patients;
- requests for medication;
- financial returns;
- requests for furniture and fittings;
- staff sickness;
- accounts of unexpected incidents in the ward.

The volume of paperwork required meant that much was done outside duty hours. The other 33–50% of senior ward nurses' administrative duties was related to patient care and was, therefore, part of their service development and monitoring role. Such duties included:

- implementing changes in ward practice, for example criteria to be used for determining when a patient was to be placed on a high level of observation;
- policies for the operation of the CPA and discharge arrangements;
- forms developed for the assessment of student nurses;
- documentation associated with staff supervision.

Time for these tasks was often reduced owing to the pressure of more routine paperwork.

Senior nurses employed a number of devices to prevent themselves being swamped by paperwork. In addition to taking work home, nurses at a number of sites divided the administrative duties between themselves. For example, G grade nurses were responsible for resource management, and F grade nurses looked after day-to-day clinical issues, including staff supervision and support. At sites where such work was delegated, nurses recognised the overlap between areas of responsibility and thus worked together on all aspects of ward management.

At four sites (A4, B7, C10 and C11), the G grade nurse was not part of the ward complement (although he or she would help if the ward was particularly busy). At one site in Region A (A4), three sites in Region B (B6, B7 and B8) and all the sites in Region C, senior staff had the services of at least a part-time ward clerk or secretary to undertake a proportion of the routine administration.

Not surprisingly, the degree to which senior nurses perceived their managerial duties to be a problem was related to whether they received administrative support. Those with support were often more tolerant of the administrative duties they performed, in contrast to those in sites where clerical support was unavailable. However, while administrative support was useful, much of the processing of the paperwork still required the input of a senior nurse, so relatively little time was released for other duties. Furthermore, many sites had a ward computer, but this was used primarily for word processing, and at only a few sites were computers networked.

Summary

Staff cover

- The number and grade of nurses on duty varied between sites irrespective of bed occupancy or other variables.
- Primary nursing was the means used to address patients' needs, but a number of logistical difficulties were highlighted.
- The difficult patient population at some sites, and peaks in demand at others, together with the volume of paperwork, meant that service development was often a reaction to events rather than part of a proactive approach to service improvement.

Staff support

- Stress and short-term staff sickness levels were increasing.
- Pressures on senior nurse time meant that clinical supervision occurred less frequently than they wished.

Barriers to effective management and leadership

The devolution of responsibilities to ward level was a double-edged sword. The greater freedom to plan and develop ward services was welcomed. The increased administrative duties, on the other hand, were disliked.

- Senior nurses' levels of responsibility varied between regions. Direct control over the ward budget was a significant influence.
- A strong link was identified between devolution, increasing paperwork and administrative duties. Grade G and F nurses saw a striking increase in the time they spent undertaking associated work, particularly office duties, over the period 1985–96.
- Senior nurses, especially in busy inner-city and district general hospital sites with over 100% bed occupancy, completed less paperwork and had more involvement in direct patient care compared with their counterparts at other sites. Pressures on other staff were significant.

Chapter 6
Caring for patients

This chapter examines the work of E and D grade staff in their role as named nurses for particular patients. It is based on an analysis of the following data:

- nurse and patient interviews;
- activity analysis;
- researcher perceptions;
- non-participant observation of shift hand-overs, MDT meetings and ward rounds;
- nurse activity and personal details, ward manager and patient questionnaires.

The named nurse role included the following activities:

- the admission of patients;
- undertaking the complete process of care: assessment; care planning, implementation and evaluating the care plan;
- attending to the patient's discharge and aftercare arrangements.

Each of these activities is discussed below.

Admission to hospital

Admission to hospital was the last resort after alternative treatment possibilities had been examined because it signified an individual's inability to cope in the community. Nurses identified four principal reasons for admission (these being consistent with findings reported in other studies, for example; Flannigan *et al.*, 1994):

1. risk of harm to self, or to others, often through lack of insight (particularly in patients with schizophrenia or other psychotic conditions);
2. self-neglect (typically patients with severe depression);
3. an inability to cope with everyday activities;
4. non-compliance with prescribed medication.

Admission to hospital usually occurred when a member of the community services, who had regular contact with an individual – community mental health nurse, social worker, consultant psychiatrist or the patient's GP – became concerned about the patient's deteriorating mental state and made a referral for hospital treatment. Such referrals resulted in planned admissions; that is, ward staff knew in advance about the patient's arrival.

A significant proportion of admissions, however, were emergency admissions (approximately 25–33% across sites, and often over 50% at busy inner-city sites), which, by definition, ward staff became aware of only shortly before the individual's arrival. Patients admitted as emergencies usually involved:

• social services staff, particularly if an individual was to be detained under the 1983 Mental Health Act or if the person had childcare responsibilities;
• police, especially if an individual had been involved in a public disturbance;
• staff in a local hospital's A&E department who were concerned about a person's mental state, particularly if he or she had been treated for self-inflicted injuries (see also Flannigan et al., 1994, who reported similar findings).

Many emergency admissions occurred at night and often when the individual was in a disturbed and distressed state. This often had a detrimental effect on the sleep of other patients. A feature of many emergency admissions was an increasing association with alcohol and drug abuse, particularly among young men aged between 18 and 25 years. This trend has been widely reported in other studies (Gournay, 1994; Johnson and Thornicroft, 1995; Mental Health Act Commission, 1995; Powell et al., 1995; Thomas et al., 1995). The abuse of alcohol and drugs made inpatients more difficult at some sites, particularly those in inner cities (see Chapter 4). In this context, the issues of risk assessment and danger were raised by ward staff.

Risk assessment and management

Although sites with more manageable populations admitted demanding patients, nursing staff at sites with difficult patient populations said
that a sustained state had resulted in a redefinition of risk. Maintaining
a safe environment had always been an issue in psychiatric wards.
Balancing the inherent unpredictability of such wards with the safety
of staff and patients was judged to be important. The task of nursing
(and other hospital) staff was to determine what was acceptable and
what was unacceptable risk. Other nursing studies draw similar
conclusions about what constitutes acceptable risk and danger (Carson
1991, 1994; Monaghan, 1993; Grounds, 1995; Moore, 1995; Potts,
1995 Alberg et al., 1996). Vinestock (1996, p. 3), for example, careful
not to overstate the level of danger in psychiatric wards, cautions that
there:

> is a small but significant risk of violence from a minority of patients.

However, nurses in the present study recounted the frequency with
which they were hit by disturbed patients. This was how one female
nurse recalled an event:

> it [being hit] does happen. I remember a case involving me not so long ago,
> where a patient had become highly irritable, because of what his voices were
> telling him to do. I went up to him to ask if he wanted a drink and he said
> 'bugger off' and lashed out, catching me on the arm. I had a big bruise on my
> arm for a few days. Those kinds of things happen fairly often.

As the patient mix became more unpredictable and difficult to
manage, the threshold for what was deemed acceptable risk had been
lowered. Severe pressure on beds and lack of suitable alternative facilities for treating severely ill people were important factors (see Chapter
4). This finding has also been referred to in other nursing studies,
including those of Carson (1991, 1994), Monaghan (1993), Grounds
(1995), Potts (1995), Moore (1995) and Vinestock (1996).

To reduce the pressure on staff and their exposure to an unacceptable level of danger, sites in Region C had introduced, as a filtering
mechanism, a pre-admission unit for emergency admissions to determine the type of ward – open or semi-secure – most appropriate for a
newly admitted patient. Here, G and F grade nurses within the unit, in
collaboration with a duty doctor, played an increasingly important
gate-keeping role. The decision to admit an individual in these
circumstances was described as a joint decision between nurse and

doctor. The development of such a filtering mechanism has also been reported in other nursing studies (Dickson, 1995; Grounds, 1995; Lipsedge, 1995; Moss, 1995; Vincent and Moss 1995; Vinestock, 1996). The patient was then admitted to the relevant ward. However, the severe demand for beds meant that the threshold had been increased to what was described as an unacceptable level, resulting in over 100% occupancies at these sites. This was a position with which senior nurses said they were unhappy. Owing to these issues, no doubt, staff at other sites said that new risk assessment procedures were being developed.

Many patients required compulsory detention under a section of the 1983 Mental Health Act, indicating that the individual was extremely ill and a risk to him or herself or to others. The high incidence of detained patients at some sites, particularly in Region C, had become established in recent years and was cited as another factor contributing to a difficult patient population (see Chapter 4). The high rates of detention have also been referred to in other studies (Barnes *et al.*, 1990; Coid, 1993; Pilgrim and Rogers, 1993; Audit Commission, 1994; House of Commons Health Committee, 1994; McDonald and Taylor, 1995; Mental Health Act Commission, 1995).

Benefits of hospitalisation

The benefits for patients of spending time in hospital were widely perceived by staff to be compromised by high bed occupancy and the difficult patient mix (see Chapter 4). The principal benefits of inpatient stays, adduced in previous studies of nursing (Flannigan *et al.*, 1994; Vinestock, 1996) were that:

- being in hospital helped to stabilise an individual's condition, so that he or she could return to everyday life, many patients thereafter continuing to receive treatment in the form of medication and ongoing support from community workers;
- hospital provided a safe haven (asylum) for patients, such an environment being important if there was a risk of self-harm or neglect;
- hospital was a place for those who were no longer able to deal with the stresses of everyday life, so-called time-out;
- the underlying causes of patients' problems could begin to be addressed in a supportive environment through contact with staff who had the skills to assess and care for those suffering from severe mental health problems.

The issues involved in admitting patients were similar across sites and are discussed below.

Admission procedures

On arrival to the ward, new patients were often confused and distressed. Therefore, they – together with relatives or friends who had accompanied them – were usually taken to a relatively quiet part of the ward to help them settle. Nursing assistants frequently carried out these tasks until a qualified member of staff arrived to undertake the formal admission procedures.

Most patients had difficulty recalling their admission to hospital, owing to the severity of their illness at the time. Some of them who could remember referred to their initial reluctance to be hospitalised. Even patients who had been admitted previously reported the fear they had before entering hospital (Altschul, 1972; Raphael, 1974; Towell, 1975; Cormack, 1976, 1983; MacIlwaine, 1983; Howard, 1992). One patient summed up her fear:

> It's not a criticism of staff, but you feel you won't leave. It's the nature of my illness. It's stigma, people see you as loony.

Ideally, a doctor and a nurse would carry out the admission procedures jointly to prevent the patient repeating basic personal information (such as name, address, next-of-kin and GP). In practice, however, there was often a delay before the doctor arrived, in which case the nurse would begin the admission procedure alone. At a number of sites, therefore, it was common practice for medical and nursing staff to undertake separate admission and assessment procedures.

After recording a new patient's personal details, the nurse would conduct an initial assessment of the patient's mental state (see below). On arrival, the doctor would also ask the patient for personal details, carry out an examination, make an initial diagnosis – pending a more thorough interview later – and, if necessary, prescribe medication.

The admitting doctor and nurse also obtained information from anyone accompanying the patient, for example relatives or a community mental health nurse, about the circumstances precipitating admission. If the patient had been admitted under a section of the 1983 Mental Health Act, the nurse checked that the paperwork was in order. Admission procedures were said to last for a minimum of 1 hour, although often lasting considerably longer.

Allocation of a new patient to a named nurse was usually to the admitting nurse or to the nurse with the smallest caseload. If the patient had been in hospital previously, he or she might ask for, or be assigned to, a particular nurse. As named nurses, grade E and D grade staff were the linchpin of individual patient care. Clinically, there were few differences in the tasks performed by E and D grade nurses, the principal one being that E grade nurses, because of their greater experience, were likely to be in charge of at least one shift per week.

The care process

A patient-centred approach to care was adopted by nurses at all sites. This involved each nurse working with a small caseload of patients to address patients' needs. Establishing a therapeutic relationship with these patients was the cornerstone of individual patient care. Devoting sufficient time to all aspects of the care process was, however, difficult to achieve in practice. The problems of patient mixes have already been referred to in Chapter 4. The issue of paperwork and administrative duties associated with care planning and the CPA are examined below. The features of therapeutic relationships are also considered.

Therapeutic relationship between named nurse and patient

The key to a successful admission is generally held to be the effectiveness of the named nurse–patient relationship (Jack, 1995; Savage, 1995; Wright, 1995). It was the named nurse who was responsible and accountable for planning and monitoring a patient's programme of care.

This relationship was important for patients in hospital. Burnard (1987a, p. 38) suggested that the aim of the relationship was 'to enter into [and understand] the perceptual world of the patient'. The success of the relationship was dependent on the following range of psychotherapeutic and interpersonal nursing skills:

- displaying empathy;
- being a good listener;
- being a good communicator;
- providing emotional support;
- being available for patients;
- valuing patients as individuals.

These are skills that have been widely and frequently reported over the years in previous nursing studies (Altschul, 1972; Towell, 1975; Burnard, 1987a, 1987b; Gijbels and Burnard, 1995).

The benefit of the nurse–patient relationship was described by one nurse in the following terms:

> You need to go on a journey with patients as they recount their problems, so that you can understand where they are coming from. You can then offer suggestions about how such difficulties can be overcome. But you need to see it from their perspective.

This echoes Burnard's (1987a, p. 38) view that:

> As another person helps us to understand our personal theory of the world, we are able to modify that theory . . . The process of exploring the theory can lead us to self disclosure and to identifying aspects of the past which are with us in the present . . . To recall and relive past experiences can often lead to a shift in perception, a change in our emotions and a resultant modification of our personal theory.

The importance of displaying empathy in their relationships with patients was frequently highlighted by ward staff. It was in this context that the patient felt that the nurse was a trustworthy person to whom the patient was likely to disclose his or her intimate personal thoughts and feelings. However, disturbing or bizarre expressions voiced by patients were not to be taken personally. As one nurse put it:

> You have to stand back from some things you may be told by patients, in order to understand why they are being said. You can't be put off by them.

Engledow (1987, p. 40) endorsed this view and added that the 'professional front' adopted by nurses 'permits the nurse to go about her duties unaffected by any disturbing feelings of pity, anger, inadequacy or insecurity.'

An important role for nurses was to listen to patients without becoming defensive or antagonistic and to understand the feelings that patients were experiencing. In the words of one nurse:

> only patients meaningfully change to create a better life for themselves, but we can assist in this process by experiencing the patients' thoughts and feelings and help them to gain self-awareness and to begin to address their problems.

The elements that comprised a therapeutic conversation between nurse and patient were the following (Burnard, 1987a):

- emphasising the present;
- focusing on feelings and keeping the patient central;
- showing empathetic understanding;
- being non-prescriptive.

Nurses initially often found it difficult to get patients to articulate their problems. The importance of developing a therapeutic relationship as a catalyst was emphasised. Three elements, in which the skills identified above were used, comprised the therapeutic relationship (Fairlie, 1992):

- establishing trust between nurse and patient;
- motivating patients;
- supporting patients.

Trust

The time spent with patients in group activities, social conversation and attending to patients' physical needs was important in developing trust between nurses and patients. Such activities were also essential prerequisites for deeper psychological help and support provided to patients during care planning (see below). Developing effective rapport with patients, important to the therapeutic relationship, was explained in three ways. The observation from a named nurse below illustrates the first way: that patients unquestioningly put their trust in those charged with caring for them (a finding noted in many previous nursing studies, for example Schutz, 1964; Danziger, 1978; Burnard, 1985; Collister, 1988; Reynolds and Cormack, 1990):

> Patients just want to get better. They trust us, the doctors and the like to help
> them get better. When they come into hospital most readily accept the sick
> role – especially if they are given medication to calm them down – and do
> whatever is necessary to get better.

Davis and Horobin (1977, p. 29) argued that being submissive, co-operative and deferential, and 'doing as you are told', were accepted aspects of hospitalisation, because patients were reluctant to 'get into trouble' and be known as a 'nuisance'. Patients were concerned that such behaviour might adversely affect the care they received.

The second explanation for nurses' rapport with patients was that early in an admission it was important for nurses to impress on patients the relatively short period of time they were likely to remain in hospital (see Tables 4.3A–D, indicating the average lengths of stay for patients interviewed). The need to demonstrate empathy was particularly important to reassure patients. Many had been very ill on admission and feared that they might never leave hospital (Burnard, 1987a; Howard, 1992). The following was a typical comment on this issue:

> You have to be honest with patients and establish the boundaries of your role. Tell them that they won't be in hospital long and that your role is to help them overcome their present crisis so that they can return home and continue to receive help in the community. They find that approach reassuring and they respect you for it.

The third rationale, an observation rarely noted in other nursing studies, was that a majority of patients were already well known to staff from previous admissions: a figure in excess of 80% was frequently mentioned (see Tables 4.3A–D). Therefore, many patients knew what to expect in hospital. As one nurse commented:

> I've seen [patient] on so many occasions it feels like we're old friends. I think that helps the relationship because the trust is there from the start.

Motivation

Motivating patients can be difficult. It requires that the nurse suspends judgement about a patient's abdication of responsibilities such as self-care and providing for the family. Burnard (1987b, p. 45) recognised that withholding judgement on another's words and actions was not easy and was perhaps the most difficult aspect of interpersonal relationships. He concluded that it was only through experience that motivation and tact could be developed by nurses:

> such skills need to be learned experientially and explored through personal involvement.

The importance of listening to patients empathetically was often emphasised. Encouraging patients to use willpower to regain control of their lives and responsibilities was important. However, it was often difficult to see positive results of the nurses' efforts. This was particularly the case early in an admission when patients were very ill and lacked insight. Patients agreed that using their willpower contributed significantly to a successful recovery: medication and support provided by nurses helped them to recognise this fact (Cormack, 1976). A nurse made the following comment:

> It's difficult when he first came to us to do anything with him. You have to wait for the medication to take effect. It's a matter of making sure that he is safe and being there when needed.

Support

Providing support to patients was said to underpin the named nurse–patient relationship. Obtaining a patient's trust and motivating them to use their willpower positively required a supportive environment between nurse and patient. This was defined as patient-centred care, which meant nurses being available for patients who gradually came to terms with the problems that precipitated the original crisis. Similar findings have been reported in previous studies: Cormack (1976), Burnard (1987a, 1987b). Engledow (1987) and Howard (1992). Responding in a caring and non-judgemental way to the feelings expressed by patients was central to this process (Burnard, 1985, 1987a, 1987b; Reynolds and Cormack, 1990). The following comments on the importance of providing support to patients were typical:

> I think probably the most important thing that I've provided for [patient] is to be there when he needs me. Just listening to his problems has been a great benefit to him, I know this because he has said so to me.

> One of the main reasons why so many people come in to the ward is that they have not been able to talk about their problems, so they bottle them up. This isn't the answer, it has to come out somewhere and that somewhere is in their deteriorating health. At least we try to provide the listening ear to patients.

> two qualities that any nurse needs to have is to be caring and to be a good listener. Without them you might as well jack it in. That's not easy at times because you have to take a lot of abuse from some of the patients. You just need to remember it's because they're ill.

Patients' emotional cues to which nurses respond

A number of emotional cues triggered responses from nurses. However, contact between nurses and patients to discuss the latter's care was infrequent, of short duration and *ad hoc* (see below). There appeared to be no clear indication of what the emotional cues were to which nurses responded. So when nurses were asked about the researchers' perceptions of nurse–patient interactions, they agreed that infrequency might appear to be the case to an outsider. They explained, however, that this was inevitable owing to the unpredictability of many interactions with patients in acute wards. Individual patients' need for support changed frequently, and other pressures on nurses' time were also significant (see Chapter 4 and the discussion below). Nevertheless, a number of cues likely to trigger a response to attend to the needs of a particular patient were identified:

- observing a patient's body language when interacting with others;
- noting whether a patient's mood or behaviour had changed recently;
- being aware of whether there had been recent changes in a patient's eating or sleeping habits.
- nurses' intuition in interpreting verbal and non-verbal cues that signified a patient's need for support (Benner, 1984; Hurst *et al.*, 1991; Hurst, 1993b).

The latter developed only through contact with patients over a number of years. The following was a typical comment expressed by a nurse:

> Much of our contact with patients appears to be *ad hoc* or unplanned. But it needs to be like that; you can't predict how some patients' mood may change during shifts or from one shift to the next. That's where ... intuition comes in; knowing when to intervene with ... It's the unpredictability of psychiatric nursing care that highlights its difference with other branches of nursing.

However, there were planned nurse–patient interactions, notably care planning (see below) although the unpredictability of mental health nursing meant that some rescheduling was often required (see Chapter 4).

Nurses acknowledged that owing to increasing pressures on their time, they tended to deal with those patients who were the most demanding or ill, and that other patients tended to be left to their own devices, especially if they were considered to pose no risk to themselves or to others (nurses' difficulty in spending sufficient time with patients is discussed in Chapters 4 and 5, and below). One nurse referred to a hierarchy of priority, dealing with the most demanding patient first. Patients also spoke of this hierarchy and either accepted it, only seeking contact with nurses if they were particularly concerned about an issue, or they were deliberately disruptive in order to secure a nurse's attention. According to one nurse:

> Yes, it is a problem [ignoring some patients]. You end up bouncing from one crisis to the next, if you're not careful. You increasingly prioritise your contact with patients: dealing with the most demanding first, while banking on others being occupied by going to OT, watching telly or amusing themselves and picking up their needs and concerns during care plan reviews. Otherwise you couldn't cope, not in a ward as busy as this.

Previous nursing studies show that nurses were not always aware of those patients who did not interact. Nurses seemed to make little use of their psychiatric skills and assess whether patients' reluctance to talk should be respected or interpreted as a non-verbal need for contact (Altschul, 1972; Towell, 1975; Benner, 1984; Hurst *et al.*, 1991; Hurst, 1993b).

Nursing care

Different nursing models for individualising patient care were used at fieldwork sites, including those of Peplau (1952), Roy (1984) and Roper *et al.* (1980), and more eclectic models that contained elements from a number of models. Despite the diversity of models, there were many similarities in the approach to patient care across sites in terms of four interrelated activities: assessment, care planning, implementation and evaluation.

Assessment

Ideally, a nursing assessment was carried out at the time of admission. If this was impossible, owing to a patient's condition, the initial assessment and care plan were completed later but were always undertaken within 72 hours of admission. The initial nursing assessment involved gathering as much information as possible about the circumstances surrounding a patient's admission. This entailed discussing with the patient the following aspects of his or her life:

- *mental state:* asking how he or she felt about the present situation, what the hopes for the future were; and why he or she needed to come into hospital;
- *psychological state:* to observe and assess how the patient interacted with others, and from talking to patients and staff;
- *social circumstances:* to identify aspects of life that might have precipitated the illness, for example housing problems, relationship difficulties or financial worries;
- *physical well-being:* to deal with any physical ailments or injuries that required immediate or ongoing attention;
- *spiritual state:* religion was significant to some patients.

Obtaining information about a patient's mental and psychological states was sometimes supplemented by carrying out psychometric tests, for example, Beck's Depressive Inventory Scale (Beck, 1976). Information obtained about these five aspects of a patient's life provided the basis of the care plan.

Care planning and implementation

The phrase 'planning for discharge' was cited as a paramount and guiding principle in the named nurse–patient relationship. This emphasised the relatively short-term nature of hospital admission to patients (also undoubtedly reflecting the severe pressure on beds at some sites; see Chapter 4).

The care plan was described as a dynamic document, which explored the different aspects of a patient's life referred to above, especially his or her mental state. Other professionals might carry out specific work with a patient: a psychologist might undertake in-depth counselling with a patient experiencing bereavement; an occupational therapist might teach skills such as cooking and other domestic activities.

Care plans have been debated in the nursing literature. McMahon (1988, pp. 39–41), for example, reported that 'In some wards the care plans were not referred to at all, while on others they were in constant use.' Moreover, care plans were 'all things to all people'. McMahon concluded that:

> Unless the care plans contain information that is useful to the reader and the information is easy to find, then the plans will be neither written nor consulted, to the detriment of individualised patient care.

MacVicar and Swan (1992, p. 39) similarly concluded about care planning in psychiatry:

> there was a wide gulf between the lofty pronouncements and what happened in the wards . . . There were no guidelines on how to record information and consequently there was considerable variation in the way the system was used. [In the literature] there was plenty of theory but nothing that could be applied directly.

Despite concerns about care plans in the literature and the present study, they were in constant use and were the mainstay of individual patient care. Care plans described:

* the patient's problems;
* activities in which the patient was involved;
* an analysis of the success of particular nursing interventions, based on discussions with the patient;
* reasons for changes to the programme of care.

Two commonly identified problems were with patients:

- complaining of difficulties in sleeping;
- expressing threats of self-harm.

Having identified the problem, an appropriate response was agreed between nurse and patient, and written in the care plan, for example monitoring sleeping over several days, perhaps aided by medication, and, for the patient threatening self-harm, to watch him or her closely using constant, one-to-one nursing.

Patients were encouraged to take an active part in the development care plans (McIver, 1991; Biehal, 1993; Rogers *et al.*, 1993; Department of Health 1994a). However, the initial assessment and care plan developed at, or soon after, admission was often produced by the nurse with little input from the patient because many patients were simply too ill to participate. For some patients, it might have been some time before they were able to contribute to care planning.

Evaluating the care plan

The care plan was used as a tool to address problems, plan an appropriate response and help evaluate the success of nursing interventions. In the examples cited above, the named nurse monitored sleep and asked the patient when it had returned to normal. With respect to self-harm, the nurse and patient examined the reasons for such expressions and explored ways of encouraging the patient to focus his or her thoughts more constructively on how present difficulties could be addressed. This might involve attending group activities organised by occupational therapists or ward staff.

Therapeutic groupwork

Three different arrangements for group activities were used:

1. off the ward, by staff in the occupational therapy department: A1, A2, B6, B7 and B8;
2. in the ward, by occupational therapy and nursing staff: A3, C9, C10 and C11;
3. in the ward, by nursing staff: A4, B5.

Nurses identified a number of benefits to patients from participating in group activities:

- providing mutual support between patients through the sharing of experiences;
- allowing patients to see that others had suffered similar difficulties prior to admission;
- helping individuals to regain confidence and motivation to come to terms with their problems;
- exposing patients to issues and situations they might encounter after they left hospital.

Groupwork also:

- helped nurses – and other hospital staff – to assess patients' progress;
- provided opportunities for nurses to engage in preventative work, assisting patients to develop coping strategies to manage their mental health problems;
- reduced the likelihood of future admissions;
- offered opportunities to observe how individual patients interacted with others.

In practice, workload pressures often dictated the frequency with which group activities occurred. Figures 6.1–6.10 and Appendix 15 show that E and D grade nurses spent little time undertaking group activities.

Any changes to a patient's programme of care were made in the light of discussions between the named nurse and the patient, and of observations made of patients during group activities. Observations were shared with colleagues during shift hand-overs and especially with the multidisciplinary care team at its weekly meeting.

Multidisciplinary working

Discussion with other hospital and community staff was another component of patient care evaluation. Especially important was the weekly MDT meeting. MDT meeting had replaced the term 'ward round', thought to emphasise medical dominance, which was no longer the case at many sites (Samson, 1995). The term 'multidisciplinary team meeting', on the other hand, suggested a meeting of equals. The medical input was only one contribution, the consensus approach to decision-making being the norm (Skelton, 1994; Geoghegan, 1995; Snowdon, 1995; Watson, 1995). The degree of consensus differed across sites, however. The MDT meeting seemed to be dominated by medical staff's views at a number of sites.

MDT meetings usually included the:

- patient;
- consultant;
- registrar or senior house officer;
- community mental health nurse;
- social worker;
- occupational therapist;
- psychologist;
- hospital mental health nurse;
- pharmacist;
- representative from the local authority housing department;
- physiotherapist.

At site A4, only the consultant, senior house officer, nurse and patient were involved. It was felt that networking and information-sharing were best undertaken outside the weekly meeting without the presence of patients. At some sites, unless issues of leave and discharge were being considered, MDT meetings were conducted without the patient. Instead, consultants preferred to see patients outside the meeting.

The MDT meeting was identified as the forum in which key decisions regarding patient care, especially changes to medication and arrangements for the discharge, were taken. At a number of sites, the MDT meeting also doubled as the CPA meeting, to discuss patients' needs after discharge (see below). Here, nursing contributions were influential owing to nurses' detailed knowledge about patients' progress.

Despite the emphasis on multidisciplinary working, many nurses said that outside the weekly MDT meeting, little multidisciplinary working occurred. Interprofessional working centred on the named nurse chasing colleagues to see whether they had acted on decisions taken by the MDT, thereby increasing the pressures on already over-burdened staff. No site had integrated multidisciplinary patient notes, although a number said that they had plans to introduce them. Hurst (1995b) identified the considerable savings in staff time that could be achieved through integrated notes.

Most patients attended the MDT meeting with great reluctance as they felt intimidated by the large number of professionals. A small number of patients even refused to attend the MDT meeting. The following two comments were typical of those made about the MDT meeting by patients:

I feel like I'm on show. I only want to see the doctor, not everybody else in the hospital!

I only want to see my consultant. Why do I have to discuss my affairs with everyone and his dog?

As indicated above, site A4 adopted a different approach to its MDT meetings. Only the consultant, senior house officer, nurse and patient were present. Patients at this site, who had experienced other hospitals, felt more comfortable with this arrangement, feeling it was more appropriate to have present only the professionals most involved in their care.

Modern nursing is a cyclical process of:

- identifying problems;
- establishing specific goals with patients to address their problems;
- implementing interventions to reach the goals;
- evaluating whether goals have been attained, including discussions among the multidisciplinary care team members;
- revisiting the problems or redefining goals in the light of the review.

Two care planning issues were raised by nurses: first, whether discussing the care plan between named nurse and patient constituted counselling; and second, the time involved in updating care plans.

Communication and counselling

Different views were expressed about whether discussions between named nurse and patient concerning the care plan constituted counselling. On the one hand, some nurses argued that, owing to a patient's relatively short hospital stay, it was inappropriate for nurses to delve too deeply into the underlying causes of a patient's illness: that was the role of others, for example psychologists. On the other hand, another group of nurses expressed disappointment that owing to pressures of work, their counselling skills were being underutilised. Instruction in such skills was limited and was acquired only subsequently by completing a recognised counselling course (see below).

Disagreement among nurses about whether nurse–patient interactions concerning care planning could be called counselling has been a common finding reported in the nursing literature over the years (Altschul, 1972; Cormack, 1976; Smith, 1988). Clarke *et al.* (1991, p. 41) explored the confusion between counselling, exercising counselling skills and exercising good communication skills. They suggested that:

One way of considering [these different skills] is to imagine a hierarchy of activities in the form of a pyramid. At the broad base lie communication skills . . . with further training and self-awareness, counselling skills can be built on to communication skills, forming the next layer up. Counselling, which requires special training and particular skills, lies at the top of the pyramid.

These authors (p. 42) defined the purposes of the different skills as:

The purpose of communication skills is to ensure appropriate social contact and interaction . . . The purpose of using counselling skills is to facilitate greater awareness and exploration of issues for the patient . . . Counselling, according to the British Association of Counselling definition, is an interaction in which one person offers another person time, attention and respect, with the intention of helping that person to explore, discover and clarify ways of living more resourcefully and toward greater well being.

Despite the apparent confusion about counselling, nurses in the present study, including those recently qualified under Project 2000, suggested that counselling and preventative activities, including educating patients about the effects of medication and what signs to look for as evidence that their mental health had begun to deteriorate, were a central focus of a nurse's work. Nevertheless, Clarke *et al.* (1991, p. 43) suggested that it was important for nurses to recognise their role limits, and to know when to refer patients to specialist counsellors:

All nurses need to have basic training in communication skills as well as basic counselling skills.

There have been other views about the nurses' counselling role. Smith (1988, p. 30) argued that there was a danger of nurses referring much of the counselling work they were capable of undertaking to others:

If nurses are not judicious, then they may find themselves on the outside looking in while others get on with the 'real' work . . . Patients leave the ward to be treated elsewhere. We see patients for medication, meals and community meetings; we are available to them during visiting and the nights . . . If a doctor wants to know what a patient is doing then it would seem natural to turn to the staff where the patient is being treated.

If nurses are perceived to have a skill deficit regarding counselling, the deficit should be addressed by, for example, counselling becoming a prerequisite for the training of mental health nurses (see also Chapters 2 and 4).

However, in the present study, nurses said that difficult patient mixes and increasing pressures on their time militated against counselling becoming a significant aspect of their work (see Chapters 4 and 5). The following encapsulated nurses' views:

> Nurses' traditional role has been in caring: providing 24 hour support and reassurance to patients. But we are increasingly being told to take on and develop the counselling side: identifying and addressing patients' underlying problems and suggesting strategies to deal with problems in the future. In practice, the patients we see in the ward and staffing levels mean that we cannot really provide a caring and counselling role. We barely cope in maintaining order in the ward to ensure a safe environment for staff and patients. If anything our role is moving further away from a counselling role to one that is more custodial, hence the emphasis on staff being C & R [control and restraint] trained.

There was general agreement among nurses that if a serious underlying problem was identified, a patient would be referred to an appropriate specialist such as a psychologist. Referrals to practitioners with the skills and time to take on a long-term role in, for example, bereavement counselling or helping a patient come to terms with childhood physical or sexual abuse was paramount. Referral also facilitated continuity of care after patients left hospital, which ward staff were unable to provide.

Site A4 proved an exception to this approach. Much of the nurse's one-to-one care planning with patients was described as counselling. Site A4 staff's emphasis on counselling was partly owing to a primary nursing philosophy, which emphasised patient-centred care and interprofessional working between hospital and community staff (Bond *et al.*, 1990). This autonomous and localised approach was adopted because of the lack of other disciplines in the hospital, in particular occupational therapists and psychologists (although such specialist services were available at another local hospital).

Inpatient services were said to be part of community services, available to users of mental health services, thus blurring the boundary between hospital and community services in the continuum of care (Department of Health, 1994a, 1996a). Ward staff regularly attended community mental health team meetings to discuss inpatients' needs and to keep abreast of recently discharged patients. There were also instances of nurses being the key worker for patients after discharge.

Nurses from all sites emphasised that as the crisis phase of a patient's illness subsided, the nature of the therapeutic relationship changed as patients became more willing and able to take a more active role in evaluating their own care plan (MacFarlane and Castledine, 1982; Grantham and Biley, 1988; Ward, 1988; Ashworth *et al.*, 1992). Changes in the relationship between nurse and patient were said to occur at the patient's pace, reinforcing the patient-centred approach to care (although pressure on beds sometimes compromised such an approach see Chapters 2 and 4).

Updating care plans

The introduction of written care plans and named nursing was widely welcomed. Such developments had contributed greatly to nurses' autonomy and the empowerment of nurses (Skelton, 1994; Snowdon, 1995; Kubsch, 1996). The importance of maintaining up-to-date care plans for disseminating patients' progress reports to nursing colleagues and other professionals was emphasised. However, owing to the difficult patient population, a permanent feature at some sites and increasingly the case at others (see Chapters 4 and 5), finding sufficient time to update the care plans was a problem. Updating required on average 30 minutes per patient per day. As a result, there was an almost overwhelming pressure to find shortcuts (McElroy et al., 1995).

As pressure on nurses to undertake more paperwork and administrative duties associated with patient care (including updating care plans) increased, their direct patient care activities suffered. Figures 6.1 and 6.2 below (see also Appendix 15) show that for E and D grade nurses respectively, over the period 1985–96, there has been a striking reduction in direct patient care:

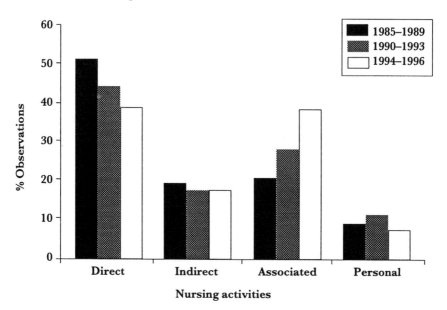

Figure 6.1 Activities undertaken by E grade nurses during recorded observations, 1985–96

For categories used in Figures 6.1–6.10, see Figure 5.1.

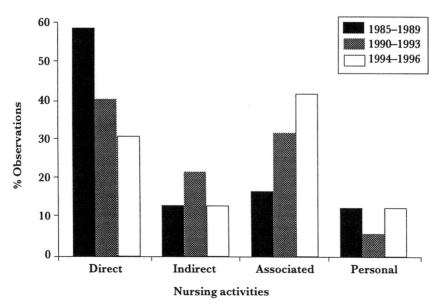

Figure 6.2 Activities undertaken by D grade nurses during recorded observations, 1985–96

- 1985–89: 52.0% and 58.2%;
- 1990–93: 44.0% and 40.4%;
- 1994–96: 39.1% and 31.2% respectively.

That is, grade E and D nurses were devoting considerably less time to direct patient care activities from 1985 to 1996. On the other hand, nurses markedly increased the time they spent in associated work, especially office duties:

- 1985–89: 20.3% and 16.5%;
- 1990–93: 27.7% and 32.1%;
- 1994–96: 37.1% and 42.3% respectively.

Figures 6.3–6.10 below provide details of activities undertaken by E and D grade nurses by:

- region;
- geographical location of hospital;
- hospital type;
- bed occupancy.

As above, the most interesting data were on nurses' time spent in direct patient care and associated work activities, especially office duties:

Region

- Grade E and D nurses in Region C devoted the most time to direct patient care activities, especially observational duties (Figures 6.3 and 6.4) – 52.3% and 45.5% – compared with their counterparts in Regions A and B: 24.5% and 32.3%, and 36.5% and 31.7% respectively.
- Grade E and D nurses in Region C assigned the least time to associated work, especially office duties (Figures 6.3 and 6.4) – 23.8% and 32.7% – compared with those in Regions A and B: 46.0% and 37.8%, and 38.2% and 45.4% respectively.

Geographical location of hospital

- Grade E nurses in inner-city locations spent the most time undertaking direct patient care activities, especially observational duties (Figure 6.5) – 43.1% – compared with those in other urban and rural locations: 38.2% and 31.8% respectively.
- Grade D nurses in other urban locations spent the least time on direct patient care activities (Figure 6.6): 17.1%, compared with 38.6% and 40.0% respectively for their counterparts in inner-city and rural locations.

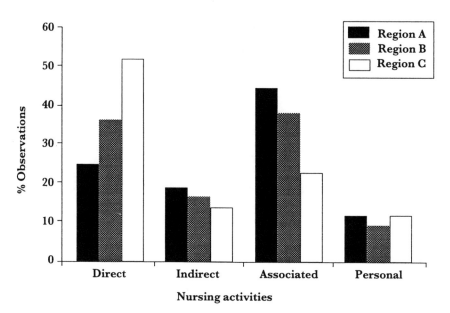

Figure 6.3 Activities undertaken by E grade nurses during recorded observations by region, 1994–96

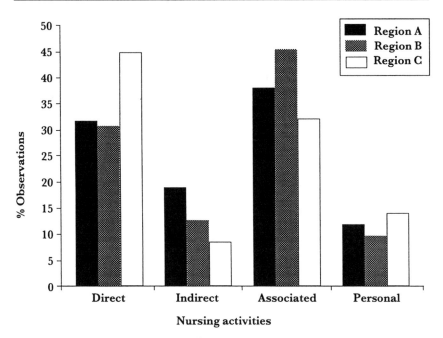

Figure 6.4 Activities undertaken by D grade nurses during recorded observations by region, 1994–96

- Grade E nurses in inner-city locations devoted less time to associated work, especially office duties (Figure 6.5): 28.7%, compared with the figures for those located in other urban and rural locations of 41.8% and 45.1% respectively.
- Grade D nurses in inner-city locations did less associated work (although they had the most time devoted to office duties; see Figure 6.6) – 36.2% – compared with their compatriots in other urban and rural locations: 60.0% and 39.1% respectively.

Hospital type

- Grade E nurses in Water Tower hospitals devoted the most time to direct patient care activities, especially observational work (Figure 6.7): 40.2%, compared with those in district general hospitals and other hospital settings – 36.7% and 36.6% respectively (although E grade nurses in district general hospitals spent more time dispensing medication to patients – 12.6% – compared with those in Water Tower hospitals and other hospital settings: 5.9% and 5.8% respectively).
- Grade D nurses in Water Tower hospitals devoted most time to direct patient care (Figure 6.8) – 44.3%– compared with their counterparts in district general hospitals and other hospital settings: 38.4% and 28.9% respectively (although D grade nurses

in district general hospitals spent more time dispensing medication to patients – 7.6%– compared with those in Water Tower hospitals and other hospital settings, with figures of 4.9% and 1.8% respectively).

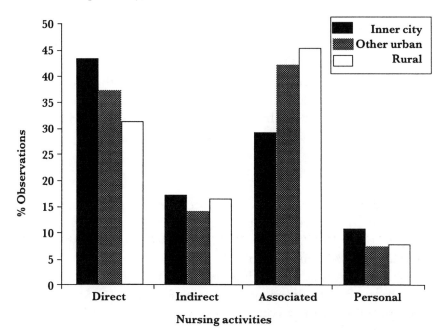

Figure 6.5 Activities undertaken by E grade nurses during recorded observations by geographical location of hospital, 1994–96

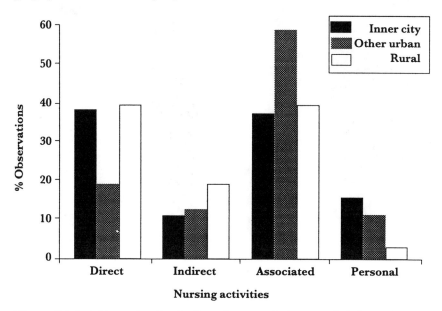

Figure 6.6 Activities undertaken by D grade nurses during recorded observations by geographical location of hospital, 1994–96

- Grade E nurses in district general hospitals spent the least time undertaking associated work (Figure 6.7): 32.6%, compared with their compatriots in Water Tower hospitals and other hospital settings – 42.5% and 39.6% respectively.
- Grade D nurses in other hospital settings spent the most time undertaking associated work (Figure 6.8), a figure of 43.7% compared with those in district general hospitals and Water Tower hospitals of 41.8% and 32.9% respectively (although D grade nurses in district general hospitals had the most time devoted to office duties – 37% – compared with those in Water Tower hospitals and other hospital settings: 28.9% and 28.2% respectively).

Bed occupancy

- Grade E nurses at sites with 100% occupancy or over devoted the most time to direct patient care, especially observational work (Figure 6.9) – 40.3% – compared with their equivalents at sites with less than 100% occupancy: 32.2%.
- Grade D nurses at sites with less than 100% occupancy devoted the most time to direct patient care (Figure 6.10) – 37.8% – compared with their counterparts at sites with 100% or over occupancy: 33.2%.

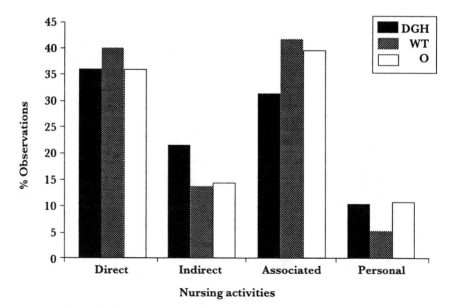

Figure 6.7 Activities undertaken by E grade nurses during recorded observations by hospital type, 1994–96

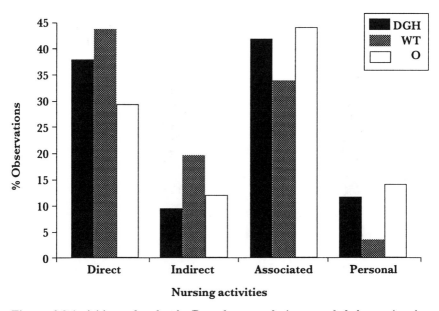

Figure 6.8 Activities undertaken by D grade nurses during recorded observations by hospital type, 1994–96

- Grade E nurses at sites with 100% occupancy or over spent the least time undertaking associated work, especially office duties (Figure 6.9), a figure of 32.5% compared with one of 40.9% at sites with less than 100% occupancy.
- Grade D nurses at sites with less than 100% occupancy spent the least time undertaking associated work (Figure 6.10) – 38.9% – but the most time for office duties – 33.2% – compared with those at sites with 100% or more occupancy, figures of 41.9% and 30.2% respectively.

In short, E grade nurses working in Region C at inner-city sites, irrespective of hospital type, with a bed occupancy of 100% or more, spent most time undertaking direct patient care activities and least time devoted to associated work, especially office duties, compared with their counterparts at other sites. The same patterns were not as strong for D grade nurses. The difficult patient populations at these sites, it would seem, required the skills of more experienced nurses. Grade E and D nurses at other sites were often under less pressure and cared for less severely ill patients. They were, therefore, able to spend more time completing paperwork than their counterparts who worked under more pressure.

One nurse summed up the care plan dilemma as follows:

> It's a problem: on the one hand it helps staff to monitor and plan a patient's care. But on the other it takes us a way from patients, so patients complain about us always being in the office doing paperwork.

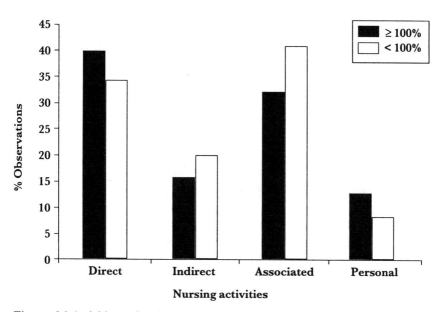

Figure 6.9 Activities undertaken by E grade nurses during recorded observations by bed occupancy level, 1994–96

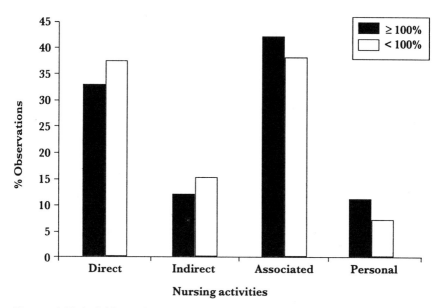

Figure 6.10 Activities undertaken by D grade nurses during recorded observations by bed occupancy level, 1994–96

Nurses generally completed the care plan after contact with the patient had finished. Nurses argued that they did not want to hinder a patient's ability to express his or her feelings, by writing comments that appeared to address a nursing agenda. Nurses might also want to comment on the patient's mental state and how the patient appeared during the interaction.

There was a potential danger of nurses selectively using information provided by patients as a short-cut, thereby recording inaccurate accounts of what was said. As noted above, owing to work pressures, particularly at busy inner-city sites (see Figures 6.5, 6.6, 6.9 and 6.10 above), nurses rarely had time to thoroughly explore all patients' concerns. The overriding need was to find shorthand ways of presenting information. However, nurses also emphasised that accurate records 'covered their backs', increasingly seen as a necessity owing to the blame and scapegoating culture prevalent within the health service. Nurses in Region C said that high-profile cases of former inpatients committing violent offences against members of the public were partly responsible for these developments. Attempting to reconcile the dilemma between undertaking direct patient care and completing paperwork increased stress and sickness among staff, particularly at sites under severe pressure (see Chapters 4 and 5).

Updating care plans also was important for liaison with others about aspects of a patient's care, for example, nursing colleagues during shift hand-over periods and with other members of the MDT. These indirect patient care activities were a significant part of the work of E and D grade nurses irrespective of region, hospital type or location and bed occupancy (see Figures 6.3–6.10 above). Typical of the comments made on this issue was the following:

> Having a care plan for patients helps us to see how he or she is progressing and what interventions are ongoing. Nevertheless, the level of detail we're expected to record, along with our other office work – answering the 'phone, speaking to relatives and doctors and writing reports for Mental Health Act Tribunals – means that you spend less and less time with patients, even if it means the quality of care has improved. It's a classic catch-22!

Two final points are worth noting on the issue of nurses' administrative duties. First, a number of sites had limited access to secretarial or IT support to help nurses record information. Second, few sites had integrated (containing the notes of all professionals involved in the patient's care) or computerised patient notes. Such developments might reduce the amount of nurses' paperwork and, therefore, the amount of liaison work (North *et al.*, 1993; Heymann and Culling 1994; Heymann *et al.*, 1994; Hurst, 1995b; Spicer *et al.*, 1995).

Other ward activities

In addition to direct patient care and administrative duties, there were indirect patient care and other associated work activities that nurses were required to undertake:

- domestic chores such cleaning and tidying (although nursing assistants or ward domestics carried out much of this work);
- errands;
- attending shift hand-overs and MDT and other ward meetings;
- answering the telephone;
- discussing patient care with ward visitors;
- teaching and assessing students.

Figure 6.1 above (see also Appendix 15) shows that, for 1994–96, E and D grade nurses respectively spent 31.4% and 34.0% of their time undertaking such activities. However, indirect and some associated tasks were identified as important aspects of patient care:

> What people forget is that there is more to working in the ward than the one-to-one work with patients. Everything that we do is important to patients. It may well be that I spend less than an hour per shift with patients, but there are many things that help a patient get better – coming out of their everyday activities, medication, interactions with other patients and even having regular meals and sleeping better.

The role of nursing assistants

Nursing assistants were valuable support to qualified staff, particularly so as pressures on nurses increased (a view also reported in other nursing studies, see for example Roberts, 1994, Workman, 1996). Figures 6.12–6.15 below (see also Appendix 15) illustrate that, in contrast to nurses, unqualified staff had relatively few administrative tasks to undertake and so spent most of their time with patients; irrespective of region, hospital type and location and bed occupancy. However, Figure 6.11 below shows that A grade nursing assistants spent less time in direct patient care between 1985–93 (72.5%) and 1994–96 (56.1%) and more time in associated work, especially office duties: 12.3% in 1985–89 compared with 13.8% in 1990–93 and 29.7% in 1994–96. These data illustrate that increasing ward pressures shifted nursing assistants' work away from direct patient care towards administrative duties, just as they had – although to a greater degree – for nursing colleagues.

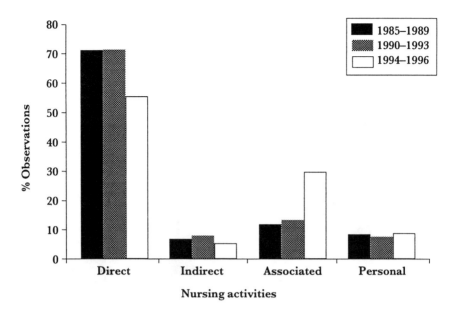

Figure 6.11 Activities undertaken by A grade nursing assistants during recorded observations, 1985–96

Notes:
1. Categories used in Figures 6.11–6.15.
D: *Direct patient care: one-to-one contact between staff and patient*: one-to-one discussions between staff and patient, care planning, assessment, comforting/controlling patient, crisis intervention; group sessions in ward; dispensing medication to patients; observations of patients; assistance with patients' personal care; escorting patient off ward for treatment; staff recreation with a patient or group of patients; ECT.
I: *Indirect patient care: discussions between staff about patients*: ward round; shift hand-overs; discussion between staff and relatives about a patient.
A: *Associated work: work that is not directly related to patient care, but is nevertheless important for the delivery of nursing care*: meetings with medical staff or other professionals, or between ward staff; office duties; teaching student nurses; domestic duties; off ward: duty nurse (Region C only); errands.
P: *Personal time*; staff breaks.
2. Obs = percentage of recorded observations.
3. Data sources: *All activities*: 1985–93, Hurst (1995a); 1994–96, present study. *Regions*: A, Yorkshire; B, Northern; C, London. *Geographical location of hospital*: IC, Inner city: A1, B7, C9, C10 and C11; OU, Other urban: A4 and B5; R, Rural: A2, A3, B6 and B8. *Hospital type*: DGH, District general hospital: A2, B7, B8 and C9; WT, Water Tower: A3, B6 and C11; O, Other hospital settings: A1, A4, B5 and C10. *Bed occupancies*: ≥ 100%: A1, B5, C9, C10 and C11; < 100%: A2, A3, A4, B6, B7 and B8.

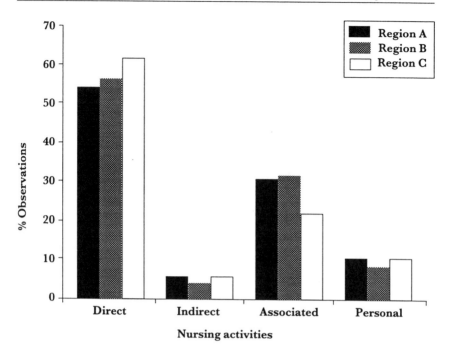

Figure 6.12 Activities undertaken by A grade nursing assistants during recorded observations by region, 1994–96

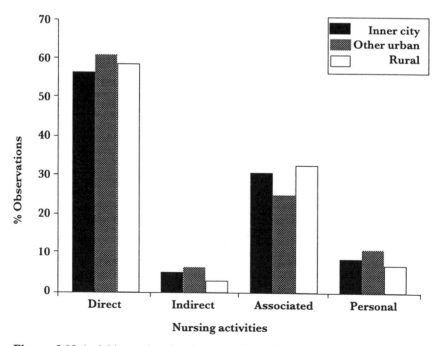

Figure 6.13 Activities undertaken by A grade nursing assistants during recorded observations by geographical location of hospital, 1994–96

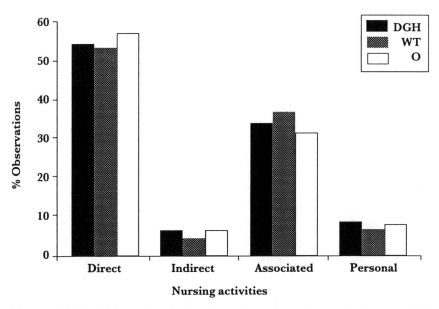

Figure 6.14 Activities undertaken by A grade nursing assistants during recorded observations by hospital type, 1994–96

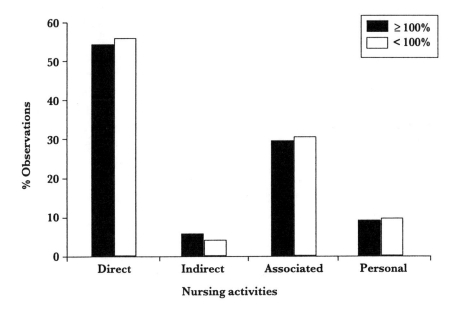

Figure 6.15 Activities undertaken by A grade nursing assistants during recorded observations by bed occupancy level, 1994–96

Figure's 6.12–6.15 show that the principal activities undertaken by unqualified staff were:

- observation work;
- working with patients;
- personal care, domestic and escort duties.

These activities were broadly similar to those reported in other studies (Roberts, 1994; Workman 1996).

Observation work

Nursing assistants were often referred to as the eyes and ears of ward staff. Nursing assistants spent most of their time making general observations of the ward situation and reporting anything significant to qualified staff. They also carried out close observation of particular patients who were deemed a potential risk to themselves or to others. One nursing assistant said:

> My job is about spending time in the ward with patients, seeing if they're OK and reporting anything strange to qualified staff. I've worked here a long time and you pick up things to look out for. You know when to report things.

Work with patients

Patient care was generally seen as the preserve of qualified staff. Nursing assistants, however, spent most time with patients, either talking to them about everyday matters or playing board games. Moreover, at a number of sites, unqualified staff had a role in patient care. This consisted of greeting and comforting new patients on admission and working closely with named nurses and patients as an associate worker. Associate workers provided support to patients and reported important developments to the named nurse or other qualified staff. The associate worker ensured that a patient always had someone with a knowledge of his or her needs in whom he or she could confide. On each shift, devising the care plan was always the remit of the named nurse. Unqualified staff, on the other hand, helped to implement the care plan:

> As the support worker to [patient] my role is to write anything that happens out of the ordinary in his care plan and to make sure he receives the agreed care in his plan. I always get a qualified member of staff to check what I've written. The main thing is to make sure that there is someone there who he knows well.

Personal care, domestic and escort duties

Unqualified staff attended to the personal care needs of patients, primarily bathing and helping patients at mealtimes (although qualified staff also carried out such duties). They also undertook domestic duties in the ward: cleaning, tidying and serving food at mealtimes (particularly if the ward did not employ domestic staff). It was mainly nursing assistants who escorted patients when attending other parts of the hospital for treatment, such as ECT, or going on social outings.

Differences across sites

There were variations in the responsibilities entrusted to unqualified staff irrespective of hospital type and location and bed occupancy. However, in Region A, nursing assistants did mostly personal care, domestic and escort duties. In Region B, on the other hand, they were involved in relatively complex aspects of nursing such as admission, care-planning and acting as an associate worker to the qualified staff, named nurse. The acquisition of level 2 NVQs was a feature in Region B sites (see below). Few grade A staff were on duty at sites in Region C.

Roberts (1994, pp. 22–3) noted that while the responsibilities undertaken by qualified staff were reasonably consistent, there was considerable variation in the responsibilities assigned to unqualified staff. This was largely owing to a lack of role clarity and pressures on nurses. Moreover, Roberts (1994) and Workman (1996) suggested that there was scope for unqualified staff to take on additional responsibilities – with further training – particularly with respect to ward and patient administration, although this idea may be resisted by the professional organisations. In practice, if nursing shortages worsen, hospital managers may have little choice but to embark on such a course. A number of other studies have questioned further whether ward staff are being used appropriately (Beardshaw and Robinson, 1990; Audit Commission, 1991; Buchan, 1992; Royal College of Nursing, 1992).

Buchan (1992) argues that the issue of cost containment has been by far the most important consideration in determining the future role of unqualified staff. As regards the introduction of vocationally trained health-care assistants (HCAs) from the late 1980s – as a replacement for traditional nursing assistant – Roberts (1994) and McKeown (1995) argued that managers have tended to perceive:

> HCAs as cheaper substitutes for qualified nurses, and plans to re-profile work-forces were raising the issue of skill substitution as a means of cost containment, usually by reducing the number of comparatively expensive qualified staff. (Roberts, 1994, p. 22)

At only two sites was a review of staff skill and grade mix under consideration. These reviews were, however, likely to see an increase in the number of qualified staff rather than a reduction. The lack of unqualified staff at sites in Region C, in contrast to Regions A and B, was reported to reflect the need for highly skilled nurses to deal with the patient mix encountered in wards (see above).

Basic and continuing education

The discussion earlier about counselling and updating care plans raised the issue about what skills nurses were taught during their initial and continuing education. Nurses were asked about the extent to which these had equipped them for their current nursing role. Table 6.1 illustrates the qualifications of staff across sites.

Table 6.1 Qualifications of staff

Qualifications

Site A1
G = 1 RMN
F = 1 RMN; BSc Psychology
E = 3 RMN × 3
D = 3 RMN × 1; SEN(MEN) × 1; RN(MEN) × 1
A = 5 Degree × 1

Site A2
G = 1 RMN; RGN; DipN; Degree
F = 1 RMN; RGN; Degree; ENB 998
E = 3 RMN × 3
D = 2 RMN × 2
A = 5

Site A3
G = 1 RMN; ENB 998
F = 1 RMN; ENB 280
E = 3 RMN × 3; ENB 998 × 1
D = 4 RMN × 3; SEN(MEN) × 1
A = 3

Site A4
G = 1 RMN; DipMan
F = 3 RMN × 3; SEN(GEN) × 1; DipSubMis × 1; ENB 612 × 1
E = 5 RMN × 5; RGN × 1; SEN(MEN) × 1; SEN(GEN) × 1; ENB 998 × 2; BSc
       Psycho-Social Behaviours x 1; DipCoun x 2; AdDipCoun × 2
D = 1 RMN
B = 1 NVQ 2
A = 1

Site B5
G = 2 RMN × 2; AdDipCoun × 1; ENB 998 × 2; ENB 553 × 1
F = 1 RMN
E = 4 RMN × 4; SEN(MEN) × 1; BA Applied Social Studies × 1;
       DipHealth (MH) × 1; DipCoun × 1
A = 1

(contd)

Table 6.1 (contd)

Qualifications

Site B6
H = 1 RMN; MBA
F = 1 RMN; ENB 998; ENB 995
E = 4 RMN × 4; ENB 998 × 2; ENB 993 × 1; ENB 995 × 1; ENB 553 × 1
D = 3 RMN × 2; SEN(MEN) × 1; DipCoun × 1
A = 4 NVQ 2 × 2

Site B7
G = 1 RMN; SEN(MEN); BSc Nursing Science; DipProf; DipCoun; ENB 998
F = 1 RMN; Degree; DipCoun; ENB 998
E = 2 RMN × 2; RGN × 1; ENB 998 × 1
D = 1 RMN
A = 3 NVQ 2 × 2

Site B8
G = 1 RMN
F = 1 RMN; SEN(MEN); DipN; CertMan; DipCoun; ENB 998
E = 5 RMN × 5; PGCE × 1; DipCoun × 2; ENB 998 × 2
D = 2 RMN × 1; RN(MEN) × 1; SEN(MEN HAND) × 1
A = 3 NVQ 2 × 2

Site C9
G = 1 RMN
F = 2 RMN × 2; SEN(MEN) × 1; BSc Health Service Management; Cert Health;
       DipCoun; ENB 998 × 1; ENB N42 × 1; ENB N46 × 1; ENB A06 × 1
E = 5 RMN × 2; RN (MEN) × 3; RGN × 1; Degree × 2; ENB 998 × 3; ENB 934 × 1
D = 3 RMN × 1; RN (MEN) × 1; SEN(MEN) × 1; Degree × 1

Site C10
G = 1 RMN; CertMan; ENB 998
F = 1 RMN; ENB 998
E = 4 RMN × 4; RGN × 1; SEN(MEN) × 1; BA Social Science × 1; ENB 998 × 2;
       ENB 934 × 1
D = 1 RN (MEN)
A = 2

Site C11
G = 1 RMN; SEN(MEN); InsCandR; AdCertLife
F = 1 RMN; ENB 998
E = 4 RMN × 3; RN (MEN) × 1; RGN × 1; ENB 998 × 2
D = 1 SEN(MEN)

Initial nurse training: RMN, State Registered Mental Nurse; RN (MEN), Registered
Nurse Mental Health (Project 2000 trained nurse with Higher Education Diploma in
Nursing); SEN (MEN), State Enrolled Mental Nurse; RGN, Registered General
Nurse; SEN (GEN), State Enrolled General Nurse; SEN (MEN HAND), State
Enrolled Mental Handicap Nurse.

(contd)

English Nursing Board (ENB) qualifications: ENB 280 Advanced HIV/AIDS; ENB 553 Care Planning; ENB 934 Care and Management of Persons with AIDS and HIV; ENB 993 Community Care; ENB 995 Control of Violent Patients; ENB 998 Teaching and Assessing in Clinical Practice; ENB A06 Certificate in Counselling; ENB N42 Principles of Mental Health Nursing and the Adult; ENB N46 Development of a Specialist Mental Health Nurse Practitioner and the Adult.

Qualifications relevant to nursing: DipCoun, Diploma in Counselling; AdDipCoun, Advanced Diploma in Counselling; DipHealth (MH), Diploma in Health Studies (Mental Health); DipN, Diploma in Nursing; DipProf, Diploma in Professional Studies of Nursing; AdCertLife, Advanced Certificate in Life Support; InsCandR ,Instructor in Control and Restraint; NVQ 2, National Vocational Qualification Level 2 in Caring.

Qualifications not specific to nursing but of some relevance; BSc Psychology, etc., first degree with some relevance to nursing; Degree, first degree of no specific relevance to nursing; MBA, Master in Business Administration ; DipMan, Diploma in Management; CertMan, Certificate in Management; CertHealth, Certificate in Health Service Management; DipSubMis, Diploma in the Management of Substance Misuse; PGCE, Postgraduate Certificate in Education.

Nurses, including staff who had only recently qualified, said that much of their initial education was largely divorced from ward work (see Chapter 2). This finding has been reported in nursing studies over many years, for example Altschul (1972), Towell (1975), Cormack (1976, 1983), Clinton (1985), Carpenter (1989), Porter (1993), Department of Health (1994a) and Gijbels (1995). Nurses who had been qualified for at least 5 years felt that their education was biased towards the physical aspects of nursing, little attention being paid to mental health issues. The dominance of the medical model, with its focus on checking signs and symptoms, accounted for this bias. The development of robust nursing models, with their emphasis on viewing patients holistically had, however, counterbalanced the dominance of the medical model (Peplau, 1952; Roy, 1984; Roper *et al.*, 1980).

This bias had been partly addressed by the introduction of Project 2000 in 1989 (United Kingdom Central Council for Nursing, Midwifery and Health Visiting, 1986, 1987). This new scheme provided recently qualified nurses with a much deeper and broader appreciation of mental health and illness, the importance of psychotherapeutic approaches and the application of communication skills in patient care (Department of Health, 1994a; Gijbels and Burnard, 1995). Using modern knowledge and skills with the current patient mix in wards, coupled with the lack of crisis management skills, anger management skills and dealing with aggressive patients, was seen as a problem by the informants (see Chapters 4 and 5). However, Project 2000-based nurse education brought new problems. The lack of practical experience in acute psychiatric wards during their education meant that newly qualified staff were largely unprepared for what they had to deal with in their wards (Department of Health, 1994a). Recently qualified nurses, therefore, often required much supervision during the initial 6–9 months of their first appointment, thereby increasing the pressures on existing staff.

The principal method of developing skills and knowledge was by reading the nursing literature. Securing time off work to attend relevant courses to develop skills often proved difficult. Cost was also an important issue, and staff were increasingly paying their own course fees. Grade G and F nurses, however, provided in-service education about nursing practice and policy developments such as the CPA. Senior nurses also had a major role in teaching and assessing student nurses. Senior staff nurses – E grades – who had completed the ENB 998 course in teaching and assessing in clinical practice also taught and assessed learners. A number of senior nurses provided training in clinical practice to medical students and junior doctors in:

- risk assessment and management;
- factors affecting the mood and behaviour of patients with particular illnesses.

The Mental Health Nursing Review Team also expressed concern at the limited availability of specific courses for mental health nurses post-registration (Department of Health, 1994a; Hamer, 1996). This was viewed with some concern by the Team. Given the recent changes to nursing practice following the introduction of the CPA, and the greater accountabilities of nurses for patient care as a result of the named nurse system, these concerns are hardly surprising (Department of Health 1994a, p. 2.2.6). In the present study, few nurses had been educated in these new aspects of nursing. The exception was the case of unqualified nursing assistants. As Table 6.1 above indicates, the skills of nursing assistants, particularly in Region B, had been developed through undertaking NVQs at level 2 in caring. At two sites – B7 and B8 – nursing assistants who had undergone NVQ preparation were renamed health-care assistants. Also, a number of nursing assistants had been encouraged to continue their education and become qualified nurses. (The role of nursing assistants is discussed in Chapter 7.)

The nursing contribution to patient care

Nurses found it difficult to isolate their contribution to patient recovery from other factors. The overall context of care was clearly important (see Chapter 4). The key to a patient's recovery consisted of finding an appropriate mix of interventions. Indeed, the trial-and-error nature of much of the work of mental health nurses is discussed in other studies (Burdock et al., 1994; Hogston, 1995; Kelsey, 1995; Mills, 1995). A typical comment made by a nurse on this issue was:

> it's like in any aspect of hospital care, a variety of things come together to make a person well; often it may not be possible to identify all the relevant things. Without an appropriate mix of things, a person won't get properly better. It's often a process of trial and error, but informed by nursing skills, knowledge and experience. If someone has been in before – many patients have – then you have some history to work from.

Bond and Thomas (1991, p. 1492) and Thomas et al. (1996) came to similar conclusions in their studies of nursing outcomes in both general and mental health nursing contexts. They noted that:

> Ascertaining whether nursing care makes a difference by using outcome measures raises methodological as well as professional issues; for example, that of separating nursing input from the inputs of other professional groups and incorporating individual patients' perspectives.

Nurses in the present study said that developments in nursing practice meant that it was now easier for them to monitor patients' progress more accurately than hitherto. The introduction of primary nursing, the system of named nurses and care-planning enabled greater consistency in the delivery of care (Department of Health, 1989, 1990b, 1993, 1994a; Mills, 1995; Watson, 1995). Such practice developments ensured a systematic approach to the delivery of care and helped to identify lines of accountability for individual patients' care. As a result, patient progress could more easily be assessed during discussions with colleagues at the weekly MDT meeting, during shift hand-overs and in more informal discussions in the ward. It was recognised that the difficult context of care prevalent at a number of sites most of the time, and at other sites less frequently, was potentially jeopardising advances made in nursing practice (see Chapters 4 and 5, and Figures 6.1–6.10 above).

Nurses emphasised that much planning for patient care was done behind the scenes, unseen by patients. Liaising and sharing information with other hospital and community staff to address patients' specific problems, for example housing and social security benefits, was also largely unseen by patients. While the approach to patient care might appear *ad hoc* to an outsider, patients received an improved quality of care through careful recording of their progress in the care plan. The researchers in this study noted that nurses were sometimes hard pressed to undertake careful recording of patients' progress, particularly at busy inner-city sites in Region C. It was difficult for them to reconcile some dilemmas:

> because of how busy the ward is and the number of staff on duty, it appears a miracle that anyone ever gets better – but they do! The nursing inputs may be spread over the week and occur at unspecified times, but patients do progress and it is possible to chart these. It helps that we know a lot of the patients who have been in before. It may appear to be chaos, but there is method in it!

Additional checks on the quality of patient care were mentioned:

- At one site, the named nurse was expected to state, in the care plan, what care and intervention patients had received in the previous 12 hours.
- The Psychiatric Monitor system was in place at other sites. This involved an annual visit by two senior nurses from another hospital, who interviewed ward staff and patients and examined nursing documentation over 2 or 3 days. They provided staff with feedback and made recommendations.
- Individual performance review systems were in place at all sites to monitor and support staff's professional development (see Chapter 5).
- Finally, representatives from the Mental Health Act Commission (for detained patients) and the Health Advisory Service carried out regular visits to all hospitals as part of their duties.

Patients' perceptions of nursing care

The majority of inpatients had nothing but the highest praise for their nursing care. This has been a consistent finding of nursing studies over the years (Altschul, 1972; Raphael and Peters, 1972; Raphael, 1974; Towell, 1975; MacIlwaine, 1983; Eriksen, 1987; Higgins, 1993). Some patients went further:

> They've [ward staff] done a lot for me. They're always there to listen to you and to talk about your problems . . . I sometimes wish that people I meet every day were as supportive and understanding as this lot [ward staff].

I can talk to them [ward staff] . . . They don't make judgements . . . It's difficult to say what it is they do to help you get better. I suppose it's being there
for you, to listen to problems and not to condemn you for ending up in here
and helping you to come to terms with what's happened . . . I don't know, but
whatever it is, it helps!

The second response above illustrated the difficulty that patients
(and nurses) had identifying precisely what aided their recovery from
an acute crisis (Bond and Thomas, 1991; Burdock et al., 1994;
Hogston, 1995; Kelsey, 1995; Mills, 1995). Many patients made the
point that the ward was often too noisy and hectic during the day to
make a positive contribution to their recovery.

Earlier, nurses identified the most important aspect of nursing care
as the therapeutic relationship established between the patient and
named nurse, a view endorsed by patients and also by the findings of
earlier nursing studies (Altschul, 1972; Towell, 1975; Cormack, 1976,
1983; Burnard, 1987a, 1987b; Howard, 1992). Patients valued their
named nurses. The term 'special nurse' was often used by patients who
emphasised the support, encouragement and advice they received
from their named nurses on matters such as illness, the effects of
medication and helping them to sort out problems before leaving
hospital.

Patients liked to feel valued and wanted and to talk to someone who
did not judge their words or actions. These nursing attributes were
important in helping patients to confront their problems. Patients
pointed out that they did speak to other ward staff, referring, for example, to the role of associate worker, who deputised when the named
nurse was not on duty.

Patients who recalled the early part of their admission reported that
they often saw their named nurse on a daily basis:

it's a bit of a blur, but I think I saw [nurse] every day. All the nurses in the
ward are very good. After a while – I've been in [hospital] for something like
two months – it drops off and I only see [nurse] odd times.

Most patients generally understood what was meant by, and that
they had, a care plan. None kept their records, and few recalled having
seen their own care plan (Department of Health, 1994a). However,
this did not concern them. Patients accepted the need for nurses – and
other hospital staff – to write about their progress as a necessary part
of being in hospital.

The one-to-one discussions that patients had with their named
nurses were viewed positively. Such sessions were seen as an important

opportunity for them to discuss how they felt with someone who understood their illness but was not judgemental. The difficulty of spending quality time with nurses was, however, identified as a specific problem. The boredom associated with hospital life was frequently mentioned by patients. Paperwork and the general pressure on staff were commonly voiced drains on staff time (see Chapter 4, and Figures 5.1–5.10 and 6.1–6.10).

Figure 6.16 below (see also Appendix 15) indicates how little time (4%) patients spent with ward staff compared with the time (28%) they spent doing nothing, watching television and undertaking personal care activities (there are no data for 1985–93):

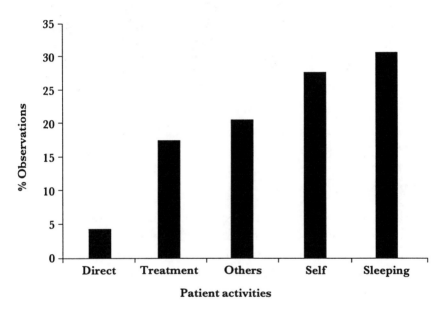

Figure 6.16 Activities undertaken by patients during recorded observations, 1994–96 only

Figures 6.17–6.20 below show the time patients spent undertaking particular activities according to region, geographical location of hospital, hospital type and bed occupancy for 1994–96.

Region

Patients in Region C spent the most time with ward staff and also the most time on their own – 5.7% and 38.4% respectively – compared with those in Regions A and B: 3.6% and 24.1%, and 3.2% and 20.4% respectively (Figure 6.17).

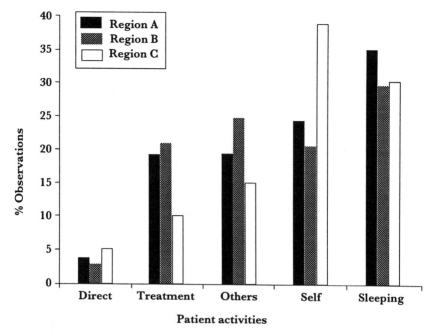

Figure 6.17 Activities undertaken by patients during recorded observations by region, 1994–96

Geographical location of hospital

Patients in inner-city locations spent the most time with ward staff and also the most time on their own (Figure 6.18), the values being 5.8% and 30.9% compared with 2.9% and 17%, and 2.9% and 27.5%, respectively, for those in other urban and rural locations.

Hospital type

Patients in other hospital settings spent the most time with staff but the least time on their own (Figure 6.19): 6% and 27.6%, compared with those in district general hospitals and Water Tower hospitals, for which the figures were 2.3% and 29.7%, and 4.6% and 31.6% respectively.

Bed occupancy

Patients at sites with 100% or over bed occupancy had the most contact with staff but also spent the most time on their own (Figure 6.20) – 4.6% and 30.8% respectively compared with those at sites with an occupancy of less than 100%: 3.5% and 23.3% respectively.

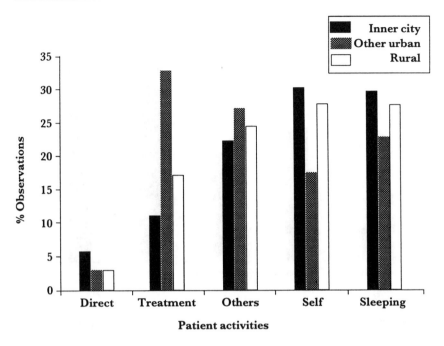

Figure 6.18 Activities undertaken by patients during recorded obervations by geographical location of hospital, 1994–96

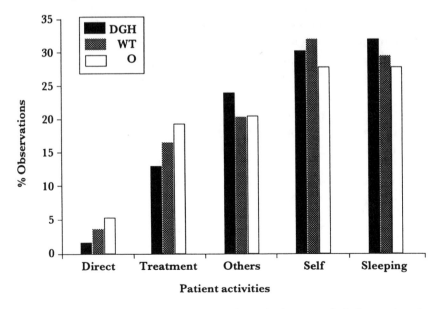

Figure 6.19 Activities undertaken by patients during recorded observations by hospital type, 1994–96

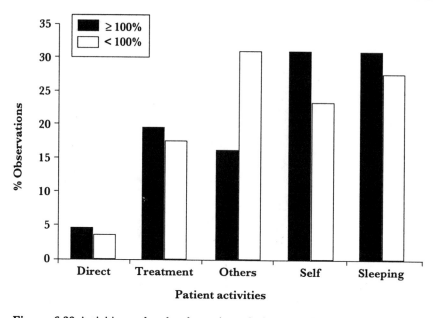

Figure 6.20 Activities undertaken by patients during recorded observations by bed occupancy level, 1994–96

Overall, patients had little contact with ward staff, irrespective of region, hospital location or type and bed occupancy. Patients spent much time on their own doing nothing, watching television or talking to other patients. Patients in inner-city sites, irrespective of hospital type, with a bed occupancy of 100% or over, especially in Region C, had the most contact with staff but also spent the most time on their own. The opposite was the case for patients in rural sites, irrespective of hospital type, with a bed occupancy of less than 100% in Regions A and B. The more demanding nature of the patient population in Region C, compared with those in Regions A and B, accounted for this pattern (see Chapter 4). The following was a typical view expressed by a patient:

> It can be difficult at times to see the nurses. They're often in the office writing or on the 'phone. You often have to deal with your problems yourself, or by chatting to fellow patients. I do have sympathy for nurses, but not being able to see them when you want is a problem – at least – for me.

Patients who offered an opinion about the one-to-one discussions with their named nurse rarely referred to them as counselling. Formal counselling was seen as the preserve of specialists such as psychologists. Patients likened the nurse's role to that of a sounding board – someone to bounce ideas off, to discuss problems with, and from whom to get advice. A patient summed up the value of her named nurse:

> she acts as a mirror, to reflect back what I say, but from a different angle. This helps to clarify my thinking and to come to terms with what's happened.

No patient mentioned medical staff fulfilling the role of counsellor. They were seen to be responsible for prescribing medication and making decisions about leave and discharge. Patients recognised that most medical decisions were based primarily on information received from nurses during the weekly MDT meeting. Many had little contact with their consultant outside this meeting. Typically, patients saw the consultant's senior house officer or registrar two or three times a week for approximately 10–15 minutes on each occasion.

Patients perceived the other professionals involved in their care – particularly medical staff – as not having the same understanding and caring attitude as nurses. Reports of studies by Towell (1975), MacIlwaine (1983) and Samson (1995) expressed similar views. This was said to be the result of lack of time that others spent with them rather than because of any lack of compassion:

> I spend all day with nurses. You build an understanding with them [doctor] only sees us once a week for a few minutes at the ward round. That's not to say he doesn't care, it's just different between patients and nurses.

Consistent with the views expressed by nurses, patients identified a number of factors that were important for helping them to get better:

- support provided by nursing and other staff;
- medication;
- being away from their everyday circumstances;
- their will.

Named nurses performed a valuable role in motivating and encouraging patients to recognise the importance of marshalling their own inner resources to positive effect (a finding consistent with those reported in other studies by Cormack (1976), Burnard (1987a, 1987b), Engledow (1987) and Bond and Thomas (1991). The following was typical of the comments made by patients:

> Nurses and doctors do a good job. The top and bottom of it is it's down to you, your own will to get better and leave [the hospital].

Detained patients tended to be less positive about their relationship with nurses owing to the imposition of treatment regimens. One detained patient su nmed up his frustration:

They said I was very ill, I accept that, but there was no need to force me to come into hospital. When you're sectioned, I imagine it's what prison is like: closely monitored, let people know what you are doing, and ask permission if you want to do anything. I don't like it and so I'm appealing against it.

Coid (1993) and the Mental Health Act Commission (1995) noted that very little attention has been given to patients detained under the 1983 Mental Health Act. Much of the literature on the legislation has focused on the mechanics of its use and its effects on services rather than patients (see also Webster *et al.*, 1987; Barnes *et al.*, 1990; Hughes, 1990; Puri *et al.*, 1992). The restrictive nature of detention was one reason why a significant proportion of those detained appealed against their section, often with the assistance of nurses (Barnes *et al.*, 1990; Coid, 1993). There is, of course, an issue about how far psychotic patients are able to judge whether their section was appropriate. Such issues are inherently difficult to explore and resolve, and are beyond the remit of the current study.

Discharge and aftercare arrangements

As patients' conditions stabilised, the issue of leaving hospital was often raised by them during a care plan review with their named nurse. The possibility of discharge was then discussed at the next MDT meeting. If discharge was considered appropriate, the CPA was activated, although certain aspects of the CPA, for example finding suitable post-discharge accommodation, could be put in place at the time of admission.

The process of discharge was similar across the study sites. Ideally, it consisted of gradually increasing lengths of leave – half a day out, an overnight stay, weekend leave, 3–4 days leave, a week's leave and so on – until discharge. After each period of leave, the named nurse and patient discussed successes and failures. This information was then fed back to colleagues at the next MDT meeting. For patients who were only in hospital for a few days, discharge was less elaborate, especially if suitable accommodation and adequate family support were available. The consultant – generally after discussion with other members of the MDT – discharged the patient and arranged an outpatient appointment.

After a number of successful periods of leave, a recommendation for discharge was made by the named nurse for a particular patient at the next MDT meeting. Nurses at a number of sites – particularly in Region C – felt that, owing to pressures on beds, some patients were sent on leave or discharged too early without sufficient preparation (see Chapter 4). This issue of discharging patients has also been noted in other studies (Hollander and Slater, 1994; Johnson and Thornicroft, 1995; Powell *et al.*, 1995).

The care programme approach

CPA was introduced in April 1991 (Department of Health, 1990b) to provide a framework for local health and social services authorities to work together – although with the health service in the lead role – to establish specific arrangements following hospital admission for the care and treatment of people in the community. Nurses said that CPA had four elements:

- A nominated *key worker* was appointed, usually either a community mental health nurse, a social worker or the patient's consultant. At site A4, ward nurses also performed this role. The role of key worker was to monitor the patient's progress after discharge.
- A full *assessment* of the patient's health and social care needs was undertaken.
- A *care plan* was drawn up by the MDT, specifying how needs were to be met.
- The care plan was *reviewed* at regular intervals.

CPA operated at all sites, although at a number it had only recently been fully implemented. The slow progress of CPA has also been noted in other studies (North *et al.*, 1993; Mental Health Foundation, 1994; Clinical Standards Advisory Group, 1995a, 1995b; Department of Health, 1995b; Malone, 1995; Social Services Inspectorate, 1995). CPA was offered to most patients where discharge was under consideration. At some sites, it was applied more selectively to individuals who met particular criteria, for example:

- patients detained under Section 3 of the 1983 Mental Health Act had a Section 117 aftercare programme in place prior to discharge;
- patients considered to be at particular risk (see section on supervision registers below).

CPA had advantages, but the related paperwork was seen as a disincentive (see Chapter 5 and Figures 6.1–6.10 above). This finding was consistent with that reported in other studies (Schneider, 1993; North *et al.*, 1993; Department of Health, 1995b; Social Services Inspectorate, 1995). CPA consisted of a checklist of actions prior to discharge. It was the named nurse who ensured that the CPA protocol was completed. His or her checklist included:

- appointing a community key worker by the MDT;
- ensuring that prescribed medication was obtained;
- making an outpatient appointment;
- organising social security benefits;
- ensuring that appropriate accommodation was available;
- considering inclusion on the supervision register.

In the meantime, the formal process of discharge was begun, as described above.

Supervision registers

Local supervision registers were introduced in April 1994 (National Health Service Executive, 1994). Their introduction was partly in response to a number of cases in which people with a history of severe mental illness had been discharged, without adequate support, and had fatally injured a member of the public; the case of Christopher Clunis was particularly significant (Department of Health, 1994b). The aim of the register is to:

- identify those people with severe mental health problems who might pose a significant risk to themselves or others;
- ensure that local services focused on those patients who had the greatest need for care and follow-up after a period of time in hospital.

Decisions to include patients on the register were made when CPA was discussed before individuals left hospital or at care programme reviews following discharge. Decisions for inclusion were made by the MDT. The formal decision to place someone on the register was ultimately that of the consultant responsible for the patient.

A patient should be included on the register, and a full risk assessment undertaken (Department of Health, 1994c), if a CPA meeting concludes that he or she is at risk in one or more of the following categories (Bottomley, 1994; Caldicott, 1994a, 1994b; Department of Health, 1994a, 1995b; Clinical Standards Advisory Group 1995a, 1995b):

- There is a risk of self harm.
- There is a risk of violence to others.
- There is a risk of self-neglect.

Few individuals were on a register at any site, and no patient interviewed knew of its existence.

Benefits and problems of CPA

Nurses said that, compared with previous discharge procedures, CPA had a number of benefits (see also North *et al.*, 1993; Social Services Inspectorate, 1995):

- *Co-ordination:* The named nurse, as care co-ordinator, was able to be more systematic about the discharge.
- *Joint working:* There was greater clarity in the roles of hospital and community staff, both before and after discharge.
- *Patient-centred approach:* Individuals were more likely to receive the aftercare and support they required.
- *Accountability:* The appointment of a named key worker was significant.
- Most important was that patients had an *aftercare plan* organised before leaving hospital.

Nurses, however, identified a major drawback with CPA: the volume of paperwork they had to complete. This involved additional written correspondence and telephoning colleagues to ensure the effective implementation of CPA. It also required nurses to spend considerable time sharing information with other professionals, organising and attending meetings, and ensuring that all the elements of a patient's care programme were in place prior to discharge. This meant that nurses were taken away from other duties. However, encouragingly, managers in a number of sites attempted to address the extra administration and meetings issue by discussing CPA at the weekly MDT meeting.

The administrative burden imposed on nurses (and other professionals) by the CPA is recognised in other studies: North *et al.* (1993, p. 3) commented on the largely 'paper driven' CPA system:

> The administration of the CPA in the hospital, and the communication it requires, places extra demands on the time of ward and medical staff.

Furthermore, Schneider (1993) and the Social Services Inspectorate (1995) noted the lack of computerised CPA records, a frequent comment expressed by nurses in the present study. On the issue of involving users and carers, North *et al.* (1993, p. 5) found that while there was widespread support for involvement, in practice CPA did not always occur (see Chapter 4).

To reduce CPA's administrative burden, ward staff suggested that it should operate at a number of levels depending on patients' needs. Indeed, the notion of the tiered CPA has also been emphasised by the recent Department of Health report *Building Bridges* (1995b). In the present study, nurses described a continuum ranging from minimal CPAs for patients with few health care needs arising from their illness, who had relatively minor support needs and were likely to remain stable, through to complex CPAs, involving the full MDT for patients with severe mental health problems, whose needs were likely to be volatile and unpredictable.

The process of implementing change through piloting a number of different CPA versions increased nurses' workloads. As nurses' familiarity increased, and the CPA procedures were refined, it was still felt that CPA generated more administrative work than did traditional approaches to hospital discharge. This problem was compounded by nurses' lack of education in CPA.

CPA and care management

Nurses spoke of their new role as CPA co-ordinators (North *et al.*, 1993; Broughton and Divall, 1994; Kingdom, 1994; Matthews, 1995). Co-ordination involved much behind-the-scenes liaison to ensure the successful implementation of the CPA for individual patients. Typical of nurses' views on CPA was the following:

> it does involve a lot of form filling. The additional work involved doesn't seem to have been accounted for, before its introduction. We have tried to address this by appointing someone to manage the process, but it still involved a lot of work for us: liaison with those involved, chasing people, arranging CPA meetings and so on.

Nurses speculated that part of CPA's problem was a lack of clarity and integration between hospital CPA procedures and local social services departments' care management systems. The former dealt with health needs and the latter with social care needs, the result of which was that nurses were undertaking aspects of discharge that they felt should have been carried out by the local authority care managers.

Patients' perspectives on discharge

Few patients were aware of what was meant by the term 'care programme approach', but patients who had been in hospital previously, and were able to recall what happened, confirmed nurses' descriptions of CPA. They did refer to the barrage of questions to which they were subjected by their named nurse prior to discharge. They also reported that their named nurse played a significant part in their discharge. The following view typified patients' views of the discharge process:

> It [discharge] seemed more involved than when I was in here last. I suppose it's better – they seemed to know what they were doing. I didn't like all the questions: what type of house I would like to live in, what I wanted to do of a day, appointments for this and that. But I suppose it's better that way than nothing.

Contrary to expectations, other than returning for outpatient appointments, or for ongoing treatment, few patients reported contact with ward nurses after discharge.

Summary

Admission to hospital

- Admission to hospital was a last resort. It signified an individual's failure to cope in the community.
- The main reason for admission was risk of self-harm or of harming others.
- Hospitalisation is about stabilising illness rather than complete recovery.
- The high proportion of emergency admissions is a feature in today's acute care.
- Risk assessment has acquired greater significance as the patient population has become more difficult to manage and the pressure on beds increased. Such pressures lead to a redefinition of acceptable risk. The introduction of pre-admission units to match available hospital resources to need was a notable development in Region C.

The care process

- A patient-centred approach was the linchpin of nursing care.
- The therapeutic relationship between the named nurse and patient was important to a successful hospital stay.
- Certain patients' emotional cues triggered a response from nurses to attend to their needs. Researchers found it difficult to see how nurses could effectively respond to patients because of the difficult patient mix at some sites. Only a small proportion seemed to have their needs adequately met.

- Nursing care consisted of assessment, care planning, implementation and evaluation.
- Two issues of concern with respect to care planning were identified: (1) whether the one-to-one discussions between named nurse and patients constituted counselling; and (2) the large amount of paperwork associated with patient care. Consequently, nurses were devoting less time to direct patient care and more time to associated work, especially office duties.
- Grade A nursing assistants provided valuable support to nurses and spent most of their time with patients. They, too, spent less time in direct patient care and more time in associated work, especially office duties. Data in this chapter illustrate that if pressures on wards increase, a shift towards administrative duties occurs.
- Difficulty in using all their skills and the lack of skills taught during initial nurse and continuing education were reported.
- Nurses and patients had difficulty isolating the nurse's contribution to patient care from those of other influences, such as medication.
- Patients had much praise for their nursing care but were critical of the boredom associated with hospital life and the lack of contact with nurses. Patients spent only 4% of their time with ward staff, compared with 28% spent doing nothing, watching television and undertaking personal care.

Discharge and aftercare arrangements

- Demand for hospital services meant that insufficient preparation for discharge had become a feature for some patients for most sites, irrespective of region, hospital location and type and bed occupancy. Insufficient preparation was a problem most of the time at inner-city sites, irrespective of hospital type, especially in Region C.
- CPA was the basis of discharge procedures but had only recently been implemented at most sites. CPA improved the co-ordination of aftercare arrangements but was paper-heavy. A lack of clarity between CPA and care management systems was reported.
- A supervision register was in place at all sites but few patients appeared in any register and none knew of its existence.

Chapter 7
Summary of findings, conclusions and recommendations

This study was commissioned by the Department of Health to investigate four main issues:

1. the patient population in acute psychiatric settings and the extent to which this has changed in recent years;
2. the nursing staff in terms of the number on duty, their grades and their qualifications;
3. the activities performed by ward staff in caring for patients;
4. patients' perceptions of their nursing care.

Patient populations

Nine sites had bed occupancies above 85% (the maximum level at which the Royal College of Psychiatrists recommends wards should operate). Of those, five sites had 100% or more occupancy, one ward having a level of 153%. Of those sites with the highest occupancies, four were located in deprived inner-city areas, three being in Region C. The patient mix in inner-city localities was classified as difficult to manage in terms of the following:

- the high proportion of patients suffering from severe mental health problems, especially schizophrenia;
- the large number of patients with a high level of dependency;
- the high percentage of patients compulsorily detained;
- the large number of patients on high levels of observation.

Such patient mixes resulted in staff finding it difficult to maintain a safe, therapeutic setting for patient care. The suitability of generic acute wards as caring environments is questionable. Acceptable risk was said to have been stretched owing to the pressure on beds, but it was unclear whether consistent and systematic risk assessment procedures were carried out. Risk assessment tools did not exist despite recent legislation on supervised discharge (Department of Health, 1995a) and the education of mental health professionals. Alberg *et al.* (1996) list risk assessment as a key issue to be addressed and offer advice on how this should be undertaken.

Acute wards primarily catered for patients requiring intensive nursing care to overcome short-lived acute psychiatric episodes. Much staff activity related to events associated with the crises of a minority of severely ill patients. Such clinical fire-fighting limited nurses' scope to implement co-ordinated, planned programmes of care for all patients (see Chapter 6).

In the light of such developments, it appeared that staff at a number of sites – particularly those with over 100% bed occupancies – were hard pressed to deal with diverse and difficult patient mixes. One consequence of pressures was an increase in stress and sickness among staff.

Basic and continuing education

Model of care

The changing role of the acute ward was at odds with the model of care with which the nurses had been made familiar. Despite the 1982 syllabus and Project 2000 emphasising counselling and nurses' involvement in the complete care process, nurses became disillusioned and suffered poor morale when they were only able to admit, stabilise and discharge rather than engage in a complete process of care. These issues might have contributed to the high turnover of staff reported at some sites. Pressures to discharge patients, in order to free beds, and weakness in community services further affected morale.

Recommendation 1: Managers and clinicians must clarify for nurses the expectations of nurses' roles at the time of recruitment for training in the nursing profession.

Recommendation 2: Managers, nurses and other clinicians must clarify for patients what they can expect when they enter hospital; that is, that, generally speaking, their condition will be stabilised and their symptoms controlled rather than that they will make a full recovery.

Skills needed

There has been a shift in the type of skills needed in acute psychiatric wards. Those needed today cover the areas of:

- crisis management;
- anger management;
- how to manage hallucinations;
- relapse management;
- co-ordinating the CPA.

An examination of the qualifications of ward staff revealed that many had acquired counselling qualifications post-registration, which they were often unable to use owing to inpatient mixes.

Concerns were expressed about the level of practical skills that newly qualified nurses brought to the ward. It was also questioned whether these nurses had sufficient contact with patients during their basic education and whether the range of experiences to which they were exposed was adequate.

Recommendation 3: In order to avoid the current mismatch between, on the one hand, the skills that nurses acquire in their initial education, and on the other, their current role in acute wards, education should encompass:

- the management of signs and symptoms;
- stabilising a patient's condition in hospital;
- co-ordinating CPA;
- facilitating the transfer of patients for care outside hospital.

Managers need to ensure that nurses' continuing education matches the clinical areas in which they work.

Activities performed by ward staff

Grade G and F nurses

Clinical supervision

A significant proportion of staff had taken sick leave in response to work pressures. Staff said that it was not uncommon for them to come in to work on their days off in order to cover for sick colleagues. Thus the need for effective clinical and managerial supervision and support becomes more important as pressures on staff increase. However, clinical supervision appeared to be *ad hoc* and unplanned.

Recommendation 4: Senior managers should examine patterns and levels of staff sickness and overtime to discover the cause and extent of the problem.

Recommendation 5: Managers and educators need to review whether the skills that nurses are taught during their initial and continuing education enable them to cope adequately with the pressures of higher bed occupancies, a higher proportion of severely ill people and a greater number of detained patients. In particular, this review should examine skills education in areas such as anger management that will enable ward staff to deal with crises, for example the threatening behaviour of some psychotic patients experiencing auditory hallucinations.

Recommendation 6: Clinical supervision should be formally recognised, carefully planned and implemented. If it is not, then there is a danger that supervision will take second place to ward demands and that opportunities for reflective practice and staff development will be missed.

Paperwork and administrative duties

The task of completing paperwork as a consequence of devolving management responsibilities to wards was identified as a particular problem for senior ward staff. Moreover, devolution has been introduced with little staff education and support. The increase in the time that G and F grade nurses spent undertaking associated work, particularly office duties, over the period 1985–96 was astonishing:

- 1985–89: 33.3% and 22.0%;
- 1990–93: 47.7% and 28.4%;
- 1994–96: 72.3% and 37.3% respectively.

As a result, the balance of senior nurses' work has shifted towards an administrative role.

At the same time, there was insufficient clarity about the nature of the nurses' clinical role and how it was to be safeguarded from administrative and management pressures. The decrease in time that G and F grade nurses spent in direct patient care has been striking over the period 1985–96:

- 1985–89: 29.0% and 44.9%;
- 1990–93: 17.3% and 34.4%;
- 1994-96: 5.7% and 22.6% respectively.

Recommendation 7: The administrative tasks undertaken by senior ward nurses should be audited to see whether they are a good use of their time, what demands on ward staff such tasks have imposed, and whether adequate administrative support has been established.

Grade E and D nurses

The significant changes in patient population at some sites were seen to be creating circumstances in which it was difficult for E and D grade nurses to implement co-ordinated, planned programmes of care for patients. Instead, they saw themselves fire-fighting – responding to the demands of the most severely ill patients and to the pressure to free beds for new admissions.

Staff nurses were clear about their role in at least three respects:

1. as a named nurse;
2. for drawing up a care plan;
3. in co-ordinating and implementating the CPA in preparation for discharge (see Chapter 6).

It is significant that these tasks focus on the *management* of care rather than the *provision* of care.

Recommendation 8: Robust pre-admission assessments need to be developed to assess and stabilise a patient's condition, either before admission to hospital or before transfer to another inpatient facility where intensive or long-term work can be undertaken.

Recommendation 9: If clinical risk assessment procedures exist, they should be more effectively disseminated and utilised. If they do not exist, they should be developed and disseminated as a matter of priority.

Recommendation 10: In view of the increasing diversity and dependency of patients cared for in acute wards, a range of care settings should be established in each locality, with staffing levels and mixes to meet patients' needs. This would include a broad spectrum of inpatient services in addition to traditional acute wards. Alternative, 24-hour nursing facilities are required for patients who need continuing longer-term care for enduring mental illnesses (Department of Health, 1996a; National Health Service Executive, 1996).

Grade E and D nurse activity

There has been a marked decrease in the time that E and D grade nurses spend in direct patient care over the period 1985–96:

- 1985–89: 52.% and 58.2%;
- 1990–93: 44.% and 40.4%;
- 1994–96: 39.1% and 31.2% respectively.

There has, on the other hand, been a striking increase in the time that E and D grade nurses spend undertaking associated work, especially office duties, between 1985 and 1996:

- 1985–89: 20.3% and 16.5%;
- 1990–93: 27.7% and 32.1%;
- 1994–96: 37.1% and 42.3% respectively.

Defensive practice

Nurses reported a growing emphasis on defensive practice and the need to cover their backs. An emerging culture of blame had become a feature of nursing at some sites and was seen to be a consequence of a relatively small number of highly publicised untoward incidents involving patients or recently discharged patients (a number of sites having been directly involved in such cases). Such incidents had reinforced the importance of written records, thereby increasing the volume of paperwork for ward staff. In any review of the administrative duties undertaken by ward staff (see Recommendation 7 above), the extent to which untoward incidents and other factors contribute to this culture of defensive practice should be acknowledged. Consideration should be given to whether nurses are appropriately equipped to write factual and succinct reports on untoward incidents.

Multidisciplinary working

The importance of multidisciplinary working was emphasised by staff. However, apart from admission and discharge procedures, such working was limited to the weekly MDT meeting. Team-building to ensure that team members understood one another's roles was never discussed. Three examples were cited by nurses to illustrate the absence of team-working:

1. With respect to patient care, nurses often spent too much time progress chasing other staff, particularly medical staff, and as a result had insufficient time to work with patients, to run groups or to provide a therapeutic environment for patient recovery.
2. Nurses were the centre of care in acute settings. Medical staff had little contact with patients and appeared to be responsible primarily for prescribing and for the formalities of admission and discharge. Moreover, therapy staff, particularly occupational therapists, did

not appear to nurses to play a core therapeutic role in patient care but were merely keeping people occupied.

3. Frequent reference was made to the nurses' new CPA care co-ordinating function. The apparent confusion in the roles performed by health service staff and local authority social services staff with respect to CPA and care management procedures was noted.

Stress and sickness, owing to pressures of work, were mentioned by ward staff as serious problems (see Recommendations 4–6 above). Participants at two feedback seminars said that if medical staff adopted a higher profile within the care team, this would reduce some of the stresses that nurses and other staff suffered. The involvement of therapy staff as core members of the ward team – rather than being located in another department – would lead to a more appropriate use of different professionals' skills and a more co-ordinated approach to patient care. Better multidisciplinary working was considered vital to reducing stress and sickness among nursing staff, especially in so far as it was associated with their isolation in the caring process.

Managers should clarify the respective roles and responsibilities of all staff working at ward level, including community personnel, in terms of delivering holistic and seamless patient care.

Recommendation 12: Managers need to ensure that sufficient time, opportunities and commitment are found to foster MDT working and development.

Recommendation 13: Integrated, multidisciplinary patient notes should be produced routinely. Among other things, they obviate the need for nurses to waste time chasing other professionals to discuss, for example, patients' aftercare.

Grade A nursing assistants

Unqualified staff had, perhaps because of workload pressures on nurses, acquired a significant nursing care role:

- operating as associate workers to named nurses;
- undertaking close observational work of patients;
- performing aspects of admission procedures and care planning.

A number of nurses, and many participants at the two feedback seminars, were concerned about whether unqualified staff had the skills and competencies to undertake the role now expected of them.

Recommendation 14: Managers should review the extent to which nursing assistants are taking on more complex aspects of mental health nursing care and the implications of this trend for both patients and staff. If nursing assistants' roles continue to develop, NVQs should be seen as one means of adequately preparing them (see Recommendation 3 above).

Patients' perceptions of nursing care

One consequence for patients of the developments described so far was that many had only passing relationships with nurses who were typically in the office writing, telephoning or dealing with unexpected incidents in the ward. This resulted in the boredom reported by many patients who, when in hospital, felt that they were often left to their own devices. Staff spent little time with patients: 4% compared with the 28% that patients spent doing nothing, watching television and undertaking personal care.

Thus patients' views corroborate those expressed by nurses about the extent to which the pressures and burdens limited nurses' direct contact with patients. Consideration should be given to relieving these nursing pressures so that nurses are able to spend more time with patients.

Recommendation 15: A detailed nursing activity analysis – different from the one undertaken in the present study – should be undertaken to consider and identify the core tasks of all grades of staff.

Recommendation 16: In order to ensure that nurses' focus is on patient care, ward clerks and nursing assistants should be used to undertake many clerical and administrative tasks and other, routine aspects of indirect patient care and associated work (see Recommendation 7 above). Investment in the appropriate information technology could also markedly reduce the amount of time that nurses spend writing patient notes.

Implications for policy and practice

This summary outlines the principal messages and implications for those agencies responsible for mental health policy and practice. Any recommendations relating to nursing theory and practice need to take account of the broader mental health picture. For example, solutions appropriate for acute settings may not be achievable without changes elsewhere. Recommendations, therefore, need to take account of skill mix, expertise, overlap and support in primary and secondary care to ensure continuity.

If appropriate skill mixes are to be achieved, separation of the skills required to care from those required to treat patients, is needed. Nurses undertake both these activities. Caring at a basic level, for example keeping patients occupied in a comfortable environment, does not require specialist (usually scarcer and expensive) nursing skills. In contrast, treating patients does require experienced nurses. If these different nursing skills are not managed, pressures on nurses working in stressful environments will increase. An overdemand for inpatient services occurs because there is an accumulation and lack of transferability of skills in acute settings. Many patients have repeat inpatient episodes because of the lack of acute mental health skills in other settings, and small numbers of patients often account for very high inpatient usage.

Issues for health authorities

- Health authorities must ensure that needs assessment, patient flow and case mix data are available to them in order to establish the level of community infrastructure and the number of inpatient beds required in the district. In view of the increasing patient dependency in acute wards, a broad spectrum of care settings and appropriate skill mix should be established in each locality. In particular, facilities are required for patients with enduring mental illness needing longer-term care.
- Health authorities need to explore individual care management as a contracting tool and move away from a dependence on block contracting. Specifications should include the required skills and approaches.
- Health authorities should explore the development of integrated care contracts with providers for people with long-term mental illness.
- Health authorities must address defensive practice in Trusts by ensuring that specifications for services include independent patient advocacy and mechanisms for recording unmet need, and must ensure their involvement in untoward incident inquiries.

Issues for health and social services authorities

- There is a need to develop integrated health and social care contracts so that care programmes across agencies are effective. A better understanding of the use of care management and how it can complement care programming should be attained by local authorities, and education events should be organised accordingly (see below).

- There is a need to ensure that specialist nursing skills are an integral part of inpatient teams and that there is continuity between inpatient and community teams. Joint appointments between hospital and community services should be explored. Skill mix studies in acute inpatient settings should address the use of social care professionals in ward teams.
- Health and social services authorities should explore the joint purchasing of services. *Building Bridges: A Guide to Arrangements for Inter-agency Working for the Care and Protection of Severely Mentally Ill People* (Department of Health, 1995b) and related reports should be used to assist this exploration.

Issues for providers

- Managers should clarify the respective roles and responsibilities of all staff, including community personnel, in terms of delivering holistic and seamless patient care. Managers need to differentiate between administrative and clinical work so that specialist nursing skills are not diluted with administrative tasks. Senior ward nurses' activities should be audited to see whether administration is a good use of their time, what demands such tasks impose and whether adequate administrative support has been established.
- Senior managers should examine the pattern and levels of staff sickness and overtime to ascertain the extent of the problem. Excessive overtime and sickness seem to be influenced by patient dependency, nursing workload, nursing establishment and grade mix.
- Skill mix and grade mix are local and national issues for which much data exist. If integrated care and treatment is to occur, staff mixes should vary according to local circumstances. Ward skill mix should not be pursued in isolation from the rest of the mental health team. A detailed analysis of nursing grade mix – different from the activity analysis undertaken in the present study – should identify the core tasks of all grades of staff.
- Clinical supervision, as a safety and competency issue, is non-negotiable and must be an integral part of ward managers' roles.
- Countering defensive practice requires that professional staff are able to share their concerns with non-executive board members. Medical and nursing management posts cannot guarantee that professional opinions and concerns are aired. Trust board

members, as a feature of clinical governance, should meet professionals as well as managers regularly and have access to user groups and patient advocacy organisations.

- Best practice in Trusts requires that the complementary roles of care management and CPA are understood and developed empirically.
- Managers, nurses and other clinicians must clarify for patients what they can expect when they enter hospital; that is, generally speaking, that their condition will be stabilised and their symptoms controlled, rather than that they will make a full recovery.
- Structures and processes are needed to assess and stabilise a patient's condition, either before hospital admission or before transfer to another inpatient facility where intensive and long-term work can be undertaken. Similarly, if clinical risk assessment procedures exist, they should be more effectively disseminated and used. If they do not exist, they should be developed and disseminated as a matter of priority.
- Managers need to ensure that sufficient time, opportunities (and commitment) are found to foster and develop MDTs.
- In order to ensure that the focus of nurses' work is patient care, ward clerks should be used to fulfil clerical and administrative tasks. An investment in the appropriate information technology could also markedly reduce the amount of time that nurses spend writing notes about patients. Integrated, multidisciplinary patient notes should be produced routinely. Among other things, these enhancements should stop nurses wasting time by chasing other professionals to discuss, for example, the aftercare of patients.

Issues for educators

- Nurse education is at the forefront of best practice and educators should, therefore, prepare nurses for changes such as care programming and supervision registers.
- The changing patient mix in acute wards requires nurses to develop a range of skills, including those relating to drug and alcohol abuse and anger management. The issue of new skills can only be addressed when a better understanding of clinical outcomes has been achieved.
- Countering defensive practices means that professional and statutory nursing bodies need to ensure that individuals are able share their concerns. Helplines and whistle-blowing protocols should be accepted as necessary supports to nurses in high-pressure environments.

- Managers and educators should review the extent to which nursing assistants take on more complex aspects of mental health nursing care, and the implications of this trend for both patients and staff. NVQs should be seen as one means of adequately preparing support staff.
- If patients are to experience continuous care, nurses and social workers must develop stronger links. Joint social work and nurse education should be part of the core curricula. Nurses should spend time with social workers in social care teams as part of their basic education, and vice versa. Trusts and local authorities should promote joint education for CPA and related topics.
- In order to avoid the current mismatch between, on the one hand, the skills that nurses acquire, and on the other, their current role in acute wards, basic education should encompass the management of signs and symptoms, stabilising patients' conditions, co-ordinating CPA and facilitating the transfer of patients to others to complete the process of care outside hospitals. Educators need to ensure also that nurses' continuing education matches the clinical areas in which they work. They need to review whether the skills taught enable nurses to cope with the pressures of higher bed occupancies, severely ill and highly dependent people, and a greater number of detained patients. In particular, this review should examine education in appropriate skills and support (such as therapeutic counselling, risk management and handling aggression) to help ward staff to deal with crises.

Appendix 1
National and
regional statistics

Beds

Nationally, the number of psychiatric beds fell by 40% between 1982 and 1991/92 (1982 = 100), and by 20% between 1988/89 and 1991/92 (1988/89 = 100). Between 1988/98 and 1991/92, the reduction was 6% in the number of short-stay beds and 35% in long-stay beds. Table A1.1 contains both national and regional figures for short- and long-stay mental illness bed changes between 1988 and 1991/92.

Table A1.1 Bed availability for mental illness: percentage change in number of available beds

Region	All beds 1982–91/92	All beds 88/89–91/92	Short stay 88/89–91/92	Long stay 88/89–91/92
All English	−40%	−20%	−6%	−35%
Northern	−29%	−14%	−9%	−23%
Yorkshire	−50%	−28%	−26%	−39%
Trent	−34%	−16%	−6%	−28%
East Anglian	−30%	−16%	−6%	−31%
NW Thames	−41%	−18%	−12%	−16%
NE Thames	−41%	−28%	−5%	−49%
SE Thames	−53%	−30%	0%	−48%
SW Thames	−39%	−18%	+2%	−30%
Wessex	−37%	−8%	+5%	−12%
Oxford	−29%	−13%	+7%	−44%
S Western	−39%	−16%	−9%	−46%
W Midlands	−38%	−17%	−3%	−36%
Mersey	−59%	−40%	−8%	−54%
N Western	−30%	−16%	−11%	−31%
SHAs	+14%	+20%	+16%	0%

Extrapolated from Department of Health bed availability data for England, 1991–92.

Short-stay psychiatric bed reductions were greater than the average in the Yorkshire, NW Thames and N Western regions (11–26%), whereas in three regions – SW Thames, Wessex and Oxford – the figure actually increased.

The numbers of short- and long-stay psychiatric beds relative to the population in each region is shown in Table A1.2. Relatively few short-stay beds were available in the Oxford, E Anglia, Wessex and SE Thames regions, and relatively large numbers in the Northern, Mersey, N Western and SW Thames regions. With regards to long-stay beds, relatively few were available in the Oxford, S Western, SE Thames and Wessex regions, and relatively large numbers in the E Anglia, NW Thames, Northern and SW Thames.

Table A1.2 Mental illness bed availability, 1991–92, excluding children and elderly

Regions	Long stay	Short stay	Population	Short stay Rate/100 000	Long stay Rate/100 000
Northern	1122	1111	2 986 934	37	37
Yorkshire	720	1057	3 535 201	30	20
Trent	1063	1375	4 692 928	29	23
E Anglian	561	502	2 136 023	24	28
NW Thames	1299	1034	3 550 591	29	37
NE Thames	1000	1301	3 750 783	34	27
SE Thames	635	1024	3 659 866	28	17
SW Thames	1779	1239	2 978 772	41	59
Wessex	538	733	2 962 329	26	18
Oxford	336	597	2 558 551	23	15
S Western	521	1154	3 289 255	35	16
W Midlands	1176	1646	5 225 395	32	23
Mersey	659	945	2 400 582	39	27
N Western	1003	1607	4 006 900	40	25

Short- and long-stay figures from Department of Health bed availability data 1991–92; population figures calculated from the *Hospital Yearbook*.

The Statistical Information Department of the Department of Health was unable to provide information on the location of short-stay psychiatric beds; this information is collated by regions and is not published nationally. However, most long-stay beds are likely to be in Water Tower hospitals, and information on the run-down of such hospitals was collected in the Survey of English Mental Illness Hospitals for the Mental Health Task Force (Table A1.3). This indicated that four or five hospitals had closed in each of the following regions since 1961: S Western, W Midlands, Yorkshire, Trent and SW

Thames. However, only one such hospital was closed in the NW
Thames, NE Thames and N Western regions, and none were closed in
the Northern region. The number of Water Tower hospitals reported
as open were as follows: 7–9 in W Midlands, Yorkshire, Trent and SW
Thames, and 3–4 in the Mersey, N Western and S Western regions.

Table A1.3 Water tower hospitals of over 100 beds

Region	Closed	Open
Northern	0	6
Yorkshire	4	8
Trent	4	7
E Anglian	3	4
NW Thames	1	6
NE Thames	1	6
SE Thames	2	6
SW Thames	4	7
Wessex	3	5
Oxford	2	5
S Western	5	4
W Midlands	5	9
Mersey	3	3
N Western	1	4

Prepared from information in the *Survey of English Hospitals*, March 1993, prepared for
the Mental Health Task Force.

In the *Hospital Yearbook*, the number of psychiatric beds is indicated
by some, but not all, district general hospitals and Trust hospitals. The
best guide to the number of such beds in district general and Trust
hospitals in each region is that the number of such beds in each type in
each region is the number of short-stay beds, as given above. However,
these short-stay bed figures may include acute psychiatric beds in
Water Tower or other hospitals.

Table A1.4 shows the number of mental illness beds and places in
England between 1982 and 1991/92. The most noticeable increases
were in private hospital beds and private mentally ill and elderly
mentally ill places, and the most notable decreases in the number of
NHS hospital beds. Nevertheless, the bulk of the long-term care of
mentally ill people still takes place in NHS hospitals.

The number of mental illness beds in private hospitals in 1992 is
shown in Table A1.5. Higher than average figures occurred in Yorkshire,
W Midlands, N Western, Mersey and SW Thames, and lower than
average ones in the Oxford, Northern and NW Thames regions.

Table A1.4 Mental illness available beds – places, England

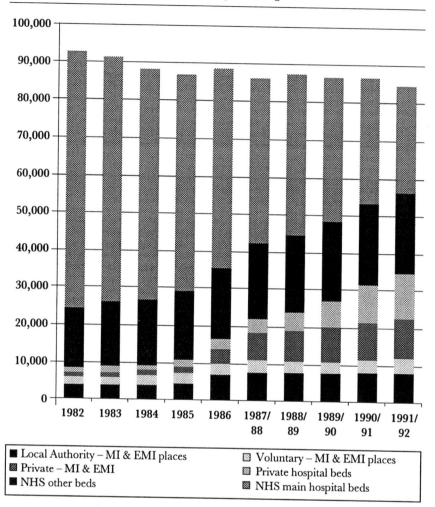

Data from Survey of English Mental Illness Hospitals, March 1993, prepared for the Mental Health Task Force; Inter Authority Comparisons and Consultancy; Mental Health Task Force; LA-RAC5, NHS-KH03, K036 returns; NB, Local Authority – EMI data only available from 1986.
MI = mentally ill; EMI = elderly mentally ill.

The vast majority of acute psychiatric care is provided in the public sector; only 7% was provided by private/voluntary sectors in 1990, and there has been little interchange between the public and private sectors (Laing, 1991). The growth in private provision that has occurred in recent years has been limited to the long-term care of mentally ill people.

Workforce

Nationally, there was an increase of 7% in the overall number of nursing

Table A1.5 Private institutions for mental illness, position at 31 March 1992; excludes children and elderly people

Region	Beds
Northern	77
Yorkshire	547
Trent	168
E Anglian	206
NW Thames	150
NE Thames	277
SE Thames	277
SW Thames	342
Wessex	213
Oxford	53
S Western	211
W Midlands	532
Mersey	391
N Western	440
All E Regions	3705

Data from 1993 edition of *Private Hospitals, Homes & Clinics Registered under s23 of the Registered Homes Act 1984.*

staff in the mental illness area of work, including community psychiatric nurses, between 1981 and 1988 (Table A1.6). The number of qualified registered staff rose by 20.8% and that of qualified enrolled staff by 3.5%, while the number of unqualified staff increased by 8.4% and the number of learners declined by 19.5%. During this period, the number of hospital nursing staff rose by 3.4%, whereas the number of community nursing staff increased by 185.2%.

Table A1.7 shows the number of nursing staff in the mental illness area of work between 1985 and 1988 by region, as well as the changes between 1985 and 1988, and 1987 and 1988. The greatest reduction in such staff between 1985 and 1988 was in the SE Thames region (32.3%), and in other regions there were relatively small changes (±7%). Between 1987 and 1988, the reduction in staff by SE Thames was 10.3%, with small changes in other regions (±4%).

Table A1.8 shows the number of qualified staff, unqualified staff and learners in the mental illness area of work in 1988 and indicates changes between 1987 and 1988. The regions with most qualified staff in post in 1988 were W Midlands, N Western and Trent. The number of qualified staff decreased between 1987 and 1988 in SE Thames and, to a much lesser extent, in Yorkshire, Mersey and NW Thames.

Table A1.6 NHS nursing staff (excluding agency) in mental illness area of work (England), at 30 September each year; whole-time equivalents

	1981	1985	1986	1987	1988	% of total	Change WTE	1981–88 (%)	Change WTE	1967–88 (%)
(a) *Overall total*	54,480	58,470	59,480	58,250	58,310	100.0	3,830	7.0	60	0.1
Qualified: total	29,200	33,140	33,760	33,040	33,390	57.3	4,190	14.4	350	1.1
Registered	18,350	20,880	21,630	21,480	22,160	38.0	3,810	20.8	690	3.2
Enrolled	10,850	12,270	12,130	11,570	11,230	19.3	380	3.5	-340	-2.9
Learners: total	8,920	8,340	8,040	7,560	7,170	12.3	-1,740	-19.5	-390	-5.1
Students	6,290	6,750	6,750	6,630	6,630	11.4	340	5.4	-10	-0.1
Pupils	2,630	1,590	1,590	930	550	0.9	-2,080	-79.1	-380	-41.1
Unqualified	16,360	16,980	16,980	17,650	17,740	30.4	1,380	8.4	90	0.5
(b) *Overall total*	54,480	58,470	58,480	58,250	58,310	100.0	3,830	7.0	60	0.1
Hospital nursing staff	53,390	56,160	56,950	55,480	55,230	94.7	1,840	3.4	-250	-0.5
Community nursing staff	1,080	2,310	2,530	2,770	3,080	53	2,000	185.2	310	11.2
Community as % of total	2.0	3.9	4.3	4.8	5.3	–	–	–	–	–

Department of Health (SM13C) *Annual Census of NHS Non-Medical Manpower*, and NHS *Worforce in England* 1990 edition.

Notes:

(1) Figures have been independently rounded to the nearest 10 whole-time equivalents. Percentages have been calculated on unrounded figures.

(2) Due to occupation coding problems, the 1987 and 1988 figures for some regions, and therefore England, are not strictly comparable with those for

Table A1.7 NHS nursing staff (excluding agency) in mental illness area of work by geographical area, at 30 September each year; whole-time equivalents

Geographical area	1985	1986	1987	1988	WTE change between 1985 and 1988	% change between 1985 and 1988	WTE change between 1987 and 1988	% change between 1987 and 1988
England	58,470	59,480	58,250	58,310	−160	−0.3	60	0.1
Northern	4,010	4,180	4,250	4,270	260	6.5	30	0.6
Yorkshire	4,610	4,710	4,710	4,590	−20	−0.4	−120	−2.6
Trent	5,360	5,600	5,650	5,670	310	5.8	30	0.5
E Anglian	2,140	2,180	2,200	2,290	150	7.0	80	3.8
NW Thames	4,510	4,650	4,460	4,360	−150	−3.3	−100	−2.2
NE Thames	4,460	4,320	4,380	4,550	90	2.0	170	3.8
SE Thames	4,060	4,070	3,060	2,750	−1310	−32.3	−310	−10.3
SW Thames	4,290	4,320	4,240	4,190	−100	−2.3	−50	−1.2
Wessex	3,380	3,430	3,500	3,550	170	5.0	50	1.4
Oxford	1,850	1,850	1,840	1,900	50	2.7	60	3.4
S Western	3,990	4,010	4,020	4,010	20	0.5	−10	−0.3
W Midlands	5,850	5,930	5,890	5,880	30	0.5	−10	−0.2
Mersey	4,070	4,140	4,050	4,020	−50	−1.2	−30	−0.8
N Western	5,320	5,510	5,450	5,670	350	6.6	230	4.2
London post-graduate special health authorities	580	580	560	610	30	5.2	50	9.3

Department of Health (SM13) *Annual Census of Non-medical manpower*, NHS Workforce in England, 1990 edition.

Notes:

(1) Figures are independently rounded to the nearest 10 whole-time equivalents (WTEs). Percentages calculated on unrounded figures.

(2) Figures include community psychiatric nursing staff.

(3) Owing to occupation coding problems, the 1987 and 1988 figures for some regions and therefore for England, are not strictly comparable with those for earlier years.

Regions with most unqualified staff in post in 1988 were N Western, Trent and W Midlands, and the largest reductions in unqualified staff between 1987 and 1988 occurred in SE Thames, Yorkshire and NW Thames.

Reductions in the numbers of learners between 1987 and 1988 took place in all regions except NE Thames, N Western and Mersey. The greatest reductions were in the S Western, E Anglia, SW Thames and SE Thames regions.

Figures provided by the Royal College of Nursing in 1992 show reductions in the number of qualified nursing posts in mental illness of 13.1% between 1987 and 1991, and 17% between 1990/91. Thus the decline in the number of qualified nursing posts in mental illness appears to be accelerating.

Table A1.8 NHS nursing staff (excluding agency) mental illness area of work by geographical area and level of qualification, at 30 September 1988; whole-time equivalents

Geographical area	Overall total		Qualified		Learners		Unqualified	
	1988	% change over 1987	1988	% change over 1987	1988	% change over 1987	1988	% change over 1987
England	58,310	0.1	33,390	1.1	7,170	−5.1	17,740	0.5
Northern	4,270	0.5	2,460	3.3	510	−8.2	1,300	−0.7
Yorkshire	4,590	−2.6	2,600	−1.3	600	−3.5	1,400	−4.5
Trent	5,670	0.4	3,250	2.7	770	−5.2	1,660	−1.1
East Anglian	2,290	4.0	1,310	5.1	220	−14.7	750	9.1
NW Thames	4,360	−2.2	2,650	−0.3	550	−9.1	1,170	−2.9
NE Thames	4,550	3.8	2,780	2.1	600	7.8	1,170	5.9
SE Thames	2,750	−10.2	1,780	−10.8	180	−10.0	790	−9.0
SW Thames	4,190	−1.3	2,400	1.2	640	−11.8	1,150	0.2
Wessex	3,550	1.4	1,890	1.9	420	−2.6	1,240	1.0
Oxford	1,900	3.4	1,130	4.3	200	−2.9	570	6.1
S Western	4,010	−0.4	2,170	2.3	410	−19.5	1,430	3.4
W Midlands	5,880	−0.1	3,380	2.1	970	−6.8	1,540	−0.2
Mersey	4,020	−0.9	2,160	−1.3	420	1.0	1,430	−0.7
N Western	5,670	4.1	3,050	3.4	600	7.9	2,020	4.1
London post-graduate special health authorities	610	9.1	410	10.3	80	10.0	130	5.0

Department of Health (SM13) *Annual Census of NHS Non-medical Manpower*, NHS Workforce in England, 1990 edition.

Notes:

(1) Includes all nurse learners undertaking pre-registration nurse training, including qualified nurses undertaking training for a second or subsequent pre-registration qualification.

(2) Figures are independently rounded to the nearest 10 whole-time equivalents (WTEs). Percentages are calculated on unrounded figures.

(3) Figures include community psychiatric nursing staff.

(4) Owing to occupation coding problems, the 1987 and 1988 figures for some regions, and therefore for England, are not strictly comparable with those for earlier years.

The number of CPNs by region between 1985 and 1988, and the percentage changes between 1985 and 1988, and between 1987 and 1988, are shown in Table A1.9. This indicates smaller increases in the number of such staff during 1988, suggesting a levelling off of the rate of increase in such staff.

Table A1.9 Community psychiatric nursing staff (excluding agency) by geographical area, at 30 September each year; whole-time equivalents

Geographical area	1985	1986	1987	1988	WTE change between 1985 and 1988	% change between 1985 and 1988	WTE change between 1987 and 1988	% change between 1987 and 1988
England	2,310	2,530	2,770	3,080	770	33.3	310	11.2
Northern	120	160	180	190	70	56.6	10	5.4
Yorkshire	170	200	220	240	70	41.2	20	10.8
Trent	220	260	290	330	110	51.6	40	14.4
East Anglian	100	110	110	120	10	21.8	10	6.2
NW Thames	160	170	160	170	10	7.0	20	12.3
NE Thames	140	140	180	210	70	50.1	30	19.5
SE Thames	160	210	150	180	20	10.9	30	17.1
SW Thames	210	210	220	230	20	10.7	10	6.5
Wessex	170	180	200	210	40	25.5	10	5.5
Oxford	110	120	120	140	30	21.9	20	14.4
S Western	140	150	200	230	90	63.8	30	15
W Midlands	240	250	290	310	70	29.2	20	6.9
Mersey	150	160	190	200	50	33.9	10	5.3
N Western	220	230	280	300	80	37.7	20	7.8
London post-graduate special health authorities	*	*	*	10	*	+	10	+

Department of Health (SM13) *Annual Census of NHS Non-medical Manpower*, NHS Workforce in England, 1990 edition.
(1) Figures are independently rounded to the nearest 10 whole-time equivalents (WTEs). Percentages are calculated on unrounded figures.
(2) These figures include all nursing staff in the community psychiatric nursing service. it is not possible to identify separately those who have undertaken post-registration training.
(3) Due to occupation coding problems, the 1987 and 1988 figures for some regions, and therefore for England, are not strictly comparable with those for earlier years.
* Less than 5
+ Numbers are so small that percentages are meaningless.

Limited information is available on other professional staff who provide services for mentally ill patients. Figures for qualified physiotherapists and occupational therapists by region in September 1988 are shown in Table A1.10. In general, the same regions had higher numbers of both, or lower numbers of both. The highest number of physiotherapists were in the W Midlands, Trent, N Western and NE Thames regions, and the lowest numbers in E Anglia, Oxford, Northern, Wessex and Mersey.

Table A1.10 Physiotherapists and occupational therapists (OTs); qualified staff in post at 30 September 1988

Region	Physiotherapists	OTs
Northern	550	230
Yorkshire	710	340
Trent	930	550
E Anglian	420	250
NW Thames	680	340
NE Thames	760	370
SE Thames	720	320
SW Thames	600	320
Wessex	550	320
Oxford	440	300
S Western	710	410
W Midlands	1080	420
Mersey	510	250
N Western	830	400
All England regions	9590	4870

Data from 1992 edition of the *NHS Workforce Statistics*.

ECT

In England, the average annual percentage change in ECT treatment per 100 000 population decreased by 5.2% between 1985 and 1990/91, the rate for 1990/91 being 220 (Table A1.11). Regional differences in 1990/91 were as follows: higher than average figures were reported in the E Anglian, Wessex, Yorkshire and N Western regions, and lower than average ones in Oxford, NE Thames, S Western, SE Thames, SW Thames and NW Thames. The greatest reductions in the use of this treatment between 1985 and 1990 were in the Northern, SW Thames, NE Thames, SE Thames and S Western regions. Mersey had increased its use of ECT between 1989/90 and 1990/91 by 18.8%, Oxford by 9.8%, E Anglia by 9.7% and SW Thames by 5.8%.

Table A1.11. ECT treatments by regional health authority 1985–1990/91, England

Regional health authority	ECT treatments per 100 000 population [1], [2]						% change between 1989/90 and 1990/91	Average annual % change 1985 to 1990/91
	1985[3]	1986[3]	1987/88	1988/89	1989/90	1990/91		
England	291	271	246	230	222	220	−1.0	−5.2
Northern	397	336	279	263	240	220	−8.4	−10.6
Yorkshire	347	359	325	328	302	276	−8.5	−4.3
Trent	312	267	250	236	231	238	2.8	−5.0
East Anglian	391	345	334	339	347	381	9.7	−0.5
NW Thames	189	203	171	180	181	177	−2.5	−1.3
NE Thames	206	183	166	156	137	123	−10.1	−9.3
SE Thames	254	239	191	185	159	171	7.4	−7.3
SW Thames	283	229	175	197	155	164	5.8	−9.9
Wessex	457	449	392	369	367	344	−6.5	−5.3
Oxford	149	133	127	109	126	138	9.8	−1.4
S Western	242	187	203	185	188	170	−9.4	−6.5
W Midlands	292	269	219	209	222	226	1.9	−4.8
Mersey	223	231	315	203	190	226	18.8	0.2
N Western	342	361	339	287	271	269	−0.8	−4.5

Data from *ECT in England*, 1991 edition.

(1) ECT treatments are based on region of treatment, whereas figures are based on region of residence.

(2) Rates are based on appropriate mid-year population estimates, e.g. 1990/91 rates are based on mid-1990 population estimates.

(3) 1985–86 data include ECT treatments administered at special hospitals, whereas KH17 data do not.

Local authority provision

Nationally, between 1980 and 1990, there was an increase of 99.6% in the total number of places in local authority staffed and unstaffed, voluntary and private homes, and an increase of 119.5% in the number of such homes (Table A1.12). The most dramatic increase in the number of places and the number of homes between 1980 and 1990 was in the private sector. Indeed, by 1990, the private sector was providing approximately 40% of places and the voluntary sector about 20%. The increase in the total number of local authority places in staffed homes was only 7.1% during the decade, and in both staffed and unstaffed homes the increase in the number of places was only 16.8%.

Table A1.12 People with mental illness: local authority staffed, unstaffed, voluntary and private homes; number of homes and number of places, England 1980–90

	Local authority						Registered homes				Total all homes	
	Staffed homes		Unstaffed homes		Total		Voluntary homes		Private homes			
	Homes	Places	Homes	Places	Homes	Places	Homes	Places	Homes	Places	Homes	Places
As at 31 March:												
1980	137	2,333	304	1,391	441	3,724	68	1,381	54	761	563	5,866
1981	146	2,467	343	1,514	489	3,981	*	*	*	*	*	*
1982	149	2,516	352	1,555	501	4,071	*	*	*	*	*	*
1983	152	2,557	375	1,616	527	4,173	118	1,603	53	764	698	6,540
1984	151	2,523	390	1,719	541	4,242	127	1,693	62	865	730	6,800
1985	156	2,563	427	1,800	583	4,363	148	1,952	102	1,219	833	7,534
1986	158	2,646	439	1,824	597	4,470	174	2,134	156	1,731	927	8,335
1987	166	2,676	476	1,957	642	4,633	165	2,103	208	2,432	1,015	9,168
1988	170 R	2,661	473	1,895	643	4,556	139	2,066	263	3,123	1,045	9,745
1989	171	2,703	522	1,994	693	4,697	162	2,325	319	3,912	1,174	10,934
1990	172	2,499	500	1,850	672	4,349	200	2,660	364	4,697	1,236	11,706
Percentage change since 1980	25.5	7.1	64.5	33.0	52.4	16.8	194.1	92.6	574.1	517.2	119.5	99.6

Data from *Residential Accommodation for Mentally Ill People and People with Learning Disabilities*, 1991 edition.

R=Revised

*Data available but not reliable.

Table A1.13 shows the regional variation in homes and places provided for mentally ill adults, and the rate per 100 000 population in 1990. The number of local authority places varied very considerably: in staffed homes, from 37 in the Southern region to 439 in Yorkshire & Humberside; and in unstaffed homes, from 66 in Inner London to 312 in Thames/Anglia. There were also considerable regional variations in voluntary and private places. The overall provision of places varied from 849 in E Midlands to 1642 in the Southern region.

Conclusions

Considerable reductions have taken place in the number of psychiatric beds over the past decade mainly, but not excessively, in long-stay beds. There were considerable regional variations in reductions in both short and long stay between 1989 and 1992, and indeed increases occurred in the number of short-stay beds in some regions.

Mirroring this decease in the number of NHS beds, there has been a marked increase in private long-stay hospital beds and private mentally ill and elderly mentally ill places. The number of private beds currently varies considerably by region.

The sparsity of recent figures makes it difficult to comment on the nursing workforce. While the number of qualified nurses, including community psychiatric nurses, rose between 1981 and 1988, there is some evidence to suggest a fall in qualified mental posts since then. The 1988 figures show considerable regional variations in qualified, unqualified and learners, but within the same region, the numbers of both qualified and unqualified nurses tend to be relatively high or relatively low. No obvious relationship was found between the number of staff and bed availability in different regions. The number of community psychiatric nurses rose considerably from 1985 to 1988, but the rate of increase appeared to be levelling off towards the end of the period.

ECT is still administered in all regions, but its use has been declining.

The number of places in local authority staffed and unstaffed homes remained fairly constant between 1980 and 1990 compared with the number of places in voluntary and particularly private homes. By 1990, about 40% of the number of places for people with mental illness in registered homes were provided by the private sector and about 20% by the voluntary sector.

Table A1.13 Homes and places provided for mentally ill adults and rate per 100 000 population and aged over 16 at 31 March 1990

Region	Local authority homes				Voluntary homes		Private homes		Total		Rate
	Staffed		Unstaffed								
	Homes	Places	Homes	Places	Homes	Places	Homes	Places	Homes	Places	
Regional totals											
Northern*	11	176	32	113	6	71	25	290	74	650	26.4
Yorks and Humberside*	27	439	57	221	8	122	45	598	137	1,380	35.0
North Western*	39	429	71	226	16	278	48	592	174	1,525	30.1
West Midlands*	19	280	48	179	20	230	35	413	122	1,102	26.6
East Midlands*	9	158	34	109	3	37	43	545	89	849	26.6
Thames/Anglia*	19	217	81	312	23	276	40	525	163	1,330	23.7
Inner London*	18	317	10	66	34	439	7	121	69	943	50.4
Outer London*	21	329	69	272	37	484	24	248	151	1,333	37.5
Southern*	2	37	42	179	33	481	62	945	139	1,642	36.2
South Western*	7	117	56	173	20	242	35	420	118	952	25.2
England total	172	2,499	500	1,850	200	2,660	364	4,697	1,236	11,706	30.7

Data from *Residential Accommodation for Mentally Ill People and People with Learning Disabilities*, 1991 edition.
*Some pre-1990 data included (see introductory notes)

Appendix 2
Trust profile

Name of NHS Trust: ....

Name and telephone number (to be contacted only in case of query):
....

Date: ....

Staff information
Hospital mental health staff establishment (WTE) at 31 March 1994:

Mental health nurses	In post	Funded establishment
Grade I	. . .	. . .
Grade H	. . .	. . .
Grade G	. . .	. . .
Grade F	. . .	. . .
Grade E	. . .	. . .
Grade D1	. . .	. . .
Grade D2	. . .	. . .
Grade C	. . .	. . .
Grade B	. . .	. . .
Grade A	. . .	. . .

Qualified grades of the following:

• Qualified outreach/link nurses	. . .	. . .
• Occupational therapists	. . .	. . .
• Physiotherapists	. . .	. . .

- Psychologists   . . .   . . .
- Psychiatrists   . . .   . . .
- Specifically employed counsellors   . . .   . . .
  (e.g. family and bereavement; please specify):

....

....

Other (please specify):

....

....

....

Community mental health staff establishment (WTE) at 31 March 1994:

	In post	Funded establishment
Community mental health nurses:	. . .	. . .
Grade I	. . .	. . .
Grade H	. . .	. . .
Grade G	. . .	. . .
Grade F	. . .	. . .
Grade E	. . .	. . .
Grade D1	. . .	. . .
Grade D2 (Enrolled Nurses)	. . .	. . .
Grade C	. . .	. . .
Grade B	. . .	. . .
Grade A	. . .	. . .

Qualified grades of the following:
- Occupational therapists   . . .   . . .
- Physiotherapists   . . .   . . .
- Psychologists   . . .   . . .
- Psychiatrists   . . .   . . .

• Other (please specify):

....

....

....

Hospital facilities at 31 March 1994

Number of acute mental health beds within general hospital   . . .

Number of acute mental health beds within private hospitals within
the boundary of your main purchasing authority   . . .

Number of acute mental health beds within long-stay (Water Tower)
hospitals   . . .

Other acute mental health facilities (please specify, with bed numbers):

....

....

....

Community facilities

Outpatients NHS facilities at 31 March 1994   . . .
Number of mental health day hospitals   . . .
Total number of mental health day hospital places   . . .
Average length of attendance (in days)   . . .
Main purpose of mental health day hospitals: . . .

....

....

Main activities undertaken in mental health day hospitals (for example, occupational therapy, art therapy, etc.):

....

....

Other community facilities, please specify (e.g. resource centre, day centre):

....

....

Total number of places   . . .
Total number of appointments   . . .
Main purpose of these facilities:

....

....

Total number of mental health secure beds:

                  low   . . .
                  medium   . . .
                  high   . . .

Additional facilities (please specify any not mentioned above):

....

....

Appendix 3
Ward environment list

Hospital
Hospital type
Ward

Lighting – bedside	1 = All beds with bedside lights
	2 = Some beds with bedside lights
	3 = No bedside lights
Lighting – ward	1 = Strip lighting throughout
	2 = Some strip lighting
	3 = No strip lighting
Windows – curtains	1 = All rooms/wards/bays with external windows curtained
	2 = Not all rooms/wards/bays with external windows curtained
Bed – curtains	1 = All beds with curtains (except beds in single rooms)
	2 = Not all beds with curtains
Floor covering	1 = Corridors and wards/rooms/bays carpeted
	2 = Ward/rooms carpeted but not corridors
	3 = Neither corridors or wards/rooms/bays carpeted
Telephones	1 = Telephones with flashing lights to replace ringing at night
	2 = Telephones that ring at night
Heating – control	1 = Heating under the control of ward staff
	2 = Heating not under the control of ward staff
Toilets	Write in the number of toilets on the ward

Toilet exits	1 = Some toilet exits directly into ward/bay
	2 = No toilet exits directly into ward/bay (toilets may exit directly into single rooms)
Baths/showers	Write in the number of baths and/or showers on the ward
Buzzers	1 = All beds fitted with buzzers
	2 = Over half of the beds fitted with buzzers
	3 = Fewer than half of the beds fitted with buzzers
	4 = No beds fitted with buzzers
Bed location	1 = Nightingale ward with or without single/double rooms
	2 = Nightingale ward and bays with or without some single/double rooms
	3 = Bays with or without some single/double rooms
	4 = Dormitory arrangement
	5 = All single or double rooms
	6 = Dormitory and some single/double rooms
Nurses' station	1 = Within Nightingale ward or in corridor outside bays
	2 = Off corridor outside bays or ward
Ward location	1 = Ground level
	2 = Above ground level
Ward noise	1 = External noise audible
	2 = External noise not audible
Smoking	1 = No smoking allowed anywhere on ward
	2 = Smoking allowed in dayroom at specified times only
	3 = Smoking allowed in dayroom at any time
	4 = Smoking only in patient's own room
	5 = Other

Admission information	1 = Written information on ward routines provided for patients on admission
	2 = Oral information on ward routines provided for patients on admission
	3 = No information on ward routines provided for patients on admission
Photographs	1 = Photographs of ward nurses on display
	2 = No photographs of ward nurses on display

Appendix 4
Ward manager
questionnaire

Hospital: Ward: Date:

Ward routines

Meal times   Breakfast   . . . . .
                     Lunch   . . . . .
                     Supper   . . . . .

Visiting times   Afternoon and evening   . . . . .
                     Afternoon only   . . . . .
                     Evenings only   . . . . .
                     Any time   . . . . .
                     Other arrangements   . . . . .

Shift times   Early day shift   . . . . .
                     Late day shift   . . . . .
                     Night shift   . . . . .

Lights on in the morning   . . . . .
Lights out at night   . . . . .
Times when nurses are not available for interview
(e.g. because of meal breaks)   . . . . .

Staff information

Staff Levels: Usual number on early shift   . . . . .
                     Usual number on late shift   . . . . .
                     Usual number on night shift   . . . . .

Internal rotation by day staff – usual number:

        From days to nights   . . . . .

        Equally on duty on days   . . . . .
        and nights

Internal rotation by night staff – usual number:

        From nights to days   . . . . .

Other nurses on duty during the day (please tick one):

Bank nurses:	Sometimes	. . . . .
	Never	. . . . .
	Always	. . . . .
Pool nurses:	Sometimes	. . . . .
	Never	. . . . .
	Always	. . . . .
Agency nurses:	Sometimes	. . . . .
	Never	. . . . .
	Always	. . . . .

Other nurses on duty during the night (please tick one):

Bank nurses:	Sometimes	. . . . .
	Never	. . . . .
	Always	. . . . .
Pool nurses:	Sometimes	. . . . .
	Never	. . . . .
	Always	. . . . .
Agency nurses:	Sometimes	. . . . .
	Never	. . . . .
	Always	. . . . .

Will there be any student nurses on the ward during the fieldwork period:

                  Yes

                  No

If yes, please indicate the days and shifts:

              . . . .

              . . . .

              . . . .

Patient information

Ward bed complement   . . . . .
Usual bed occupancy   . . . . .

Average length of stay   . . . . .
Usual number of patients sectioned:
        Section 2   . . . . .
        Section 3   . . . . .
        Section 4   . . . . .
        Section 5(2)   . . . . .
        Section 5(4)   . . . . .
        Section 37   . . . . .
        and other section (please specify) . . . .
        . . . .
        . . . .

Usual number of patients suffering from:
        (1)   Schizophrenia   . . . . .
        (2)   Affective (mood) psychosis   . . . . .
        (3)   Depressive disorders   . . . . .
        (4)   Anxiety states   . . . . .
        (5)   Dementia   . . . . .
        (6)   Eating disorders   . . . . .
        (7)   Personality disorders   . . . . .
        (8)   Drug problem   . . . . .
        (9)   Alcohol/substance abuse   . . . . .
        (10)   Child abuse   . . . . .
        (11)   Social problems   . . . . .
        (12)   Other (please specify) . . . .
        . . . .

        Usual number of patients on different observation levels:
            Observation 1   . . . . .
            Observation 2   . . . . .
            Observation 3   . . . . .
            Observation 4   . . . . .

        Are care plans used on the ward?   Yes
                                                 No

        Standards of care on the ward (please tick one):
            Written standards
            Verbal standards
            No formal standards

Number of ECT sessions available per week (please tick one):
> One
> Two
> None available
> Other (please specify) . . . .

Usual number of patients from this ward receiving
ECT treatment each week   . . . . .

Number of occupational therapy sessions available per week:
> Mornings   . . . . .
> Afternoons   . . . . .

Usual number of patients from this ward who go to
occupational therapy each week:
> Mornings   . . . . .
> Afternoons   . . . . .

Are other therapies provided off the ward?   Yes
                                                                    No

If yes, please list the type of therapy, and the usual number
of patients from this ward who attend each week:

Therapy	Patients per week
. . . .	. . . .
. . . .	. . . .
. . . .	. . . .

Appendix 5
Fieldwork plan

1. Contact will be made with the Chief Executive/Unit General Manger in each fieldwork location, and permission sought to carry out fieldwork in one ward. Meetings will be arranged with senior nurse managers and the ward manager, and fieldwork dates agreed.

2. Ethical committee approval will be sought in each location.

3. Fieldwork will be undertaken over a period of 5 days. All the procedures described below will be piloted in the two locations in which the qualitative work was undertaken, and practices/instruments amended as required.

   i) A patient list will be prepared, and the nurse in charge of the ward asked whether any patients should be excluded from participating in the research because of their medical condition. The remaining patients will be randomly selected and ordered according to their selection. Patients will be approached in selection order, and their consent sought until we have obtained five patients prepared to participate in the project. These patients will be asked to complete a *pro forma* and be interviewed. They will also be informed that they will be observed over certain periods of time.

   ii) Duty rotas will be used to prepare a list of nurses on duty during the fieldwork period. We will ask each nurse to complete a *pro forma*, and to be interviewed. Nurses will be asked about their activities with regard to patients in general, and also specifically about the five selected patients. Those who have been in post for a number of years will be asked to compare present demands with those that were made on them 5 years ago.

iii) Nurses and patient activity will be recorded during one night shift, and during one early and one late day shift. Activities performed by all the nurses on duty will be recorded. In addition, the five selected patients will be observed.

iv) Profiles of the district, hospital and ward will be obtained at each location, and the ward manager will be interviewed about ward routines and practices.

v) Information departments in each location will be asked for any details they have of staff in post and of inpatients on the selected ward during the first week in September 1988.

vi) On the last day of fieldwork in each location, or as soon afterwards as can be arranged, a meeting will take place to discuss the experiences of the research team at the location.

vii) The material obtained from each location will be collated, analysed and written up. When all the fieldwork in one region has been completed, a feedback session for managers and nursing staff will be arranged.

Appendix 6
Ward manager and nurse interview questions

What is the age range of patients on this ward?
Do you have patients of different ethnic origins on this ward?
How many of each?

How many patients have been on mental health wards before their present hospitalisations?

To what extent are patients transferred to other wards?
If so, what are the reasons?

How many patients are readmitted within 2 weeks of discharge (other than those for whom a bed has been reserved)?

Would you please describe the hand-over on this ward? (See additional questions)

What is the usual grade mix of staff on the different shifts?

Are there any differences between day and night shifts?
If so, what are these?

(Probe: Management issues)

Which grades of staff rotate from days to nights or vice versa?

Do you operate the '24-hour nurse responsibility system' for named nurses?

If so, how does this work in practice?

Would you please describe the admission and assessment process?
Prompt:

  admission policy
  length of time for assessment
  determination of observation level
  allocation to key worker

How would you describe the patient care provided on this ward?
Prompt:

  philosophy
  patient involvement in care planning
  principal objectives
  review/assess objectives
  evaluation of nursing input

What nursing practice is used on this ward during the day?
Prompt:

  how are ward staff organised?
  who allocates work?
  how is the duty rota compiled (e.g. for the ward as a whole, or
  within teams)?
  who has nursing accountability for patient care?
  who is responsible for writing the nursing notes?
  who liaises with the medical staff?

How do nurses prioritise their work?

Would you please describe the ward round
Prompt:

  who is involved?
  how often do these take place?
  do the nurses and other professionals 'report back' on the patients?
  does the patient attend?

Do you see the medical staff on the ward at other times?
Prompt:

  how often?
  what for?
  do patients usually see the doctor (other than at the ward round)?

Do nurses ever work under the supervision of someone other than a more senior member of the ward nursing staff? Whom? Why?

Which other professionals are involved with your patients? In what ways? Does anyone co-ordinate this input? Who does this?
Prompt:

> OTs
> psychotherapists
> psychologists
> CPNs
> other health workers
> social workers
> housing department
> other local authority departments

Would you describe the discharge process?
Prompt:

> who makes the decision?
> involvement of other professionals (see above)
> links between hospital and community

Whose responsibility is it to ensure that appropriate community care is available when the patient leaves hospital? Who is responsible for the patient's community care after discharge?

What changes have occurred during the past 5 years:

- in the patient population?
- in the staffing levels?
- in the demands on nurses?
(Probe: increase in sickness levels – reasons)
- in the nursing practice used on the ward by day and by night?
- in facilities within the hospital for mental health patients?
- in facilities in the community for mental health patients?

Hand-overs

Who is involved during hand-overs?

How many nurses are on the ward during hand-overs?

Who takes the lead at hand-overs?

What is discussed during hand-overs?
(Probe: Patient care; unexpected incidents)

How long do they generally take?

Is any documentation referred to during hand-overs?

Is any paperwork associated with hand-overs?
If so, what does this involve?

To what extent are hand-overs to and from night staff different from
hand-overs from early to late day shifts?
If so, how?

Questions for qualified nurses on night duty

Admission process

Do you get many admissions during the night?
If so, who refers them?
What are people generally admitted for?

What is your role regarding people who are admitted at night?

Whose decision is it to admit someone?
Would he/she see a doctor at this time?
If so, what do they do?

What paperwork is required?
Do you prepare a care plan at this stage?

What were the principal criteria used to determine whether to admit
the patient?

To what extent have the types of patients on the ward changed in
recent years?
(Probe: Increased violence on ward; increase in the length of inpatient stay; increase in referrals from police; homelessness; breakdown in community support systems)

Assessment Process

Do you begin the assessment process with those admitted during the night?
If so, what is involved?

What are the main purposes of this?
(Probe: Determination of level of observation; developing a care plan)

Who else is involved?

What is their role?
(Probe: Involvement of relatives; negotiation with patient)

What is the end result of this process?
(Probe: Development of a care plan)

Do you do any assessments on those already in hospital?
If so, what does this involve?

Inpatient care

Once the person has been admitted and assessed, what are the principal tasks that you undertake in caring for the patient?

What is/are the purpose of this/these?
(Probe: Seek clarification about talking to patient, especially if this is linked to a therapy/counselling role of nurse; content of conversation; developing a relationship; how long these conversations last; how often you spend time with patients each week; administering medication, dealing with side-effects and reporting back to the doctor; tending to patients' physical care needs; observing patients (what do you do when observing those on level 1 and 2 observation?); recreation with patient; skills teaching/treatment advice/relaxation sessions)

How much time do you actually spend with patients?

How is the remainder of your time spent?

Is there a lot of paperwork/office work involved?
If so, describe this.

How much time does this take during an average shift?

To what extent does this type of work prevent you spending more time with patients?

Have you worked on days in the past?
If so, are there any differences between the day and night shifts?
If so, what are they?

Are hand-overs to and from night staff different from hand-overs from early to late day shifts?
If so, how?

Have there been any significant changes introduced to do with patient care in the past 5 years or so?
If so, what are they?

Have they affected the care that you provide for the patient?

Working with others

Do you generally see other professionals on the ward at night?
If so, who and for what purpose?

To what extent are there multidisciplinary meetings to discuss the patients' care?

What is the purpose of these?
Is the patient usually involved?
If so, why?
If not, why?

Do you see relatives at night?
If so, for what reasons?

Discharge process

Are people discharged at night?
If so, what does this involve?

Has CPA been offered to any of your patients?

Has this approach been used with any of your patients?

Who was appointed key worker?
Have you had any feedback from the patients or key workers about it?

Whose responsibility is it to ensure that the discharge arrangements are undertaken?
(Probe: A particular individual; a team – hospital and/or community)

To what extent will you be involved with the patient after he/she leaves hospital?

To what extent is this responsibility passed on to someone else?
If so, who?

How is this process managed?

Training

When did you undertake your training?

To what extent do you feel that it has equipped you to undertake the nursing task required of you for patients?

Did you receive instruction in making relationships with patients/listening/dealing with aggression/control and restraint?

To what extent do you have the opportunity to undertake further training to update your skills?

Have you taken any in the last 5 years or so?
If so, what?
If not, why?

What skills do you use in your work?

Do you have 'specialist' skills that you use with patients?
If so, what are these?
(Probe: For example, bereavement counselling)

Did you obtain these as part of your initial training, or subsequently?

Have there been any significant changes in nursing practice in recent years?
If so, what are they?

What impact has it had on your work?

Are you involved in the assessment/teaching of students/juniors?

If so, what is involved?

Questions for unqualified nurses on night duty

Admission process

Do you get many admissions during the night?
If so, what are people generally admitted for?

Are you involved in the admission process?
If so, what is your role?

Are you required to do any paperwork?
If so, what is your role?

To what extent have the types of patient on the ward changed in recent years?
(Probe: Increased violence on the ward; increase in the length of inpatient stay; increase in referrals from police; homelessness; breakdown in community support systems)

Assessment process

Do you begin the assessment process during the night?
If so, are you involved and what do you do?

Do you assess people who are already in hospital?

Are you involved?
If so, what do you do?

What is/are the main purposes of this?

Are you required to do any paperwork?
If so, what is involved?

Who else is involved?

What is their role?

(Probe: Involvement of relatives; negotiation with patient)

What is the end result of this process?
(Probe: Development of a care plan)

Inpatient care

Once the person has been admitted and assessed, what are the principal tasks that you undertake in caring for the patient?

What is/are the purpose of this /these?

(Probe: Seek clarification on: talking to patient – especially if this is linked to the therapy/counselling role of nurse; content of conversation; developing a relationship; how long these conversations last; how often you spend time with patients each week; administering medication; dealing with side-effects and reporting back to the doctor; tending to patients' physical care needs; observing patients (what do you do when observing those on level 1 and 2 observation?); recreation with patient; skills teaching/treatment advice/relaxation sessions)

How much time do you actually spend with patients?

How is the remainder of your time spent?

Are you required to undertake any paperwork/office work?
If so, describe what is involved?

How much time does this take during an average shift?

To what extent does this type of work prevent you spending more time with patients?

Have you worked on days in the past?

Are there any differences between the day and night?
If so, what are they?

Have there been any significant changes introduced to do with patient care in the past 5 years or so?
If so, what are they?

How have they affected the care that you provide for the patient?

Working with others

Do you generally see other professionals on the ward at night?
If so, who?

What is the purpose?

To what extent are there multidisciplinary meetings to discuss patients' care?

What is the purpose of these?
Is the patient usually involved?
If so, why?
If not, why?

Do you see relatives at night?
If so, for what reasons?

Discharge process

Are people discharged at night?
If so, are you involved?

What do you do?

Are you required to undertake any paperwork?
If so, what is involved?

To what extent will you be involved with the patient after he/she leaves hospital?

To what extent is this responsibility passed on to someone else?
If so, who?

How is this process managed?

Training

To what extent do you have the opportunity to undertake further training to update/extend your skills?

Have you undertaken any in the past 5 years or so?
If so, what?

If not, why?

What skills do you use in your work?

Do you have any specialist skills that you use with patients?
If so, what are these?
(Probe: For example, bereavement counselling)

Have there been any significant changes in nursing practice in recent years?
If so, what are they?

What impact has it had on your work?

Questions for qualified nurses who are not named nurses

Admission process

Are you involved in the admission process?
If so, what is your role?

What are the main reasons for hospitalising individuals?
(Probe: Provision of a safe environment; management of illness)

What are the principal criteria used to determine whether to admit a person?

Are patients on section treated differently?
If so, how?

To what extent have the types of patients on the ward changed in recent years?
(Probe: Increased violence on ward; increase in the length of inpatient stay; increase in referrals from police; homelessness; breakdown in community support systems)

Assessment process

Are you involved in the assessment process?
If so, what is/are the main purposes of this?
(Probe: Determination of level of observation; developing a care plan)

What is your role in this process?

What is the end result of this process?
(Probe: Development of a care plan)

To what extent are those patients on a section treated differently?
(Probe: Observation level)

Inpatient care

How would you define the nursing care that you provide?
(Probe: 'Nursing philosophy'; purpose; leadership issues)

Once a person has been admitted and assessed, what are the specific tasks that you undertake with the patient?

What is/are the purpose of this/these?
(Probe: Seek clarification on: talking to patient – especially if this is linked to the therapy/counselling role of nurse; content of conversation; developing a relationship; how long these conversations last; how often you spend time with patients each week; administering medication, dealing with side-effects and reporting back to the doctor; helping with ECT; tending to patients' physical care needs; escorting patient off the ward; observing patients (what do you do when observing those on level 1 and 2 observation?); group sessions involving patient (relaxation/discussion); recreation with patient; and skills teaching/treatment advice/relaxation sessions)

What is meant by?:
Behaviour modification therapy (seclusion, time-out)
Cognitive therapy
Bereavement counselling
Counselling skills and how distinguished from counsellor
Psychotherapy
Psycosocial intervention

Are any of these therapies practised on this ward?

Do you practise any of them?

Are patients ever referred to others off the ward for any of these therapies?

How do nurses set appropriate boundaries to their professional, therapeutic input?

If you practise any of the above therapies, how were you taught to do so (peers, clinical supervision, courses, reading)?

Would you say you were experienced in dealing with any of the following: loss, depression, anxiety, confusion, dementia?

To what extent are patients involved in decisions affecting their care?

What kind of areas are the patients involved in?

What is their input into reports on their condition at the ward round?

Examples.

Are advocates for patients ever sought?

Do you think advocates for patients have a role to play?

How much time do you actually spend with patients?

How is the remainder of your time spent?

Are you required to do much paperwork/office work?
If so, describe this.

What paperwork is associated with patient care?

What other paperwork/office work is there?
How much time does this take during an average shift?

To what extent does this type of work prevent you spending more time with patients?

Do you work on nights?
If so, how does this differ from working on days?
(Probe: Time with patients)

To what extent are the hand-overs to and from night staff different from the hand-overs from early to late day shifts?

Have there been any significant changes introduced to do with patient care in the past 5 years or so?

If so, what are they?

How have they affected the care that you provide for the patient?

Working with others

To what extent do you meet with the doctor to discuss patients' care?

What is the purpose of such meetings?

Is the patient usually involved?

If so, why?

If not, why?

How do your nursing notes relate to patients' medical notes?

To what extent do you meet with other professionals to discuss patients' care?

Who else is involved?

What is the purpose of such meetings?

Is the patient usually present?

If so, why?
If not, why?
(Probe: Housing department personnel; DSS personnel about benefits)

To what extent do you meet with relatives to discuss patient care?

To what extent is/are any of the nursing interventions under the clinical supervision of someone else?
If so, who?
What are the interventions involved?

What is the purpose of such supervision?

Is such practice common?
If so, how long has it been operating?

Discharge process

How do you determine when a patient is ready for discharge?

Whose decision is it?
(Probe: Doctor; multidisciplinary team; patient; community team; hospital team)

What is your role in the process?

Has CPA been offered to any of your patients?

Has this approach been used with any of your patients?

How does it differ from previous discharge arrangements?

Who was appointed key worker?

Have you had any feedback from patients or key workers about it?

How are the hospital and community services co-ordinated?

Do you have networks in the community?
If so, what are they?

How do they link with the hospital?

Whose responsibility is it to ensure that patients receive the appropriate community care?

To what extent will you be involved with the patient after he/she leaves hospital?

To what extent is this responsibility passed on to someone else?
If so, who?

How is this process managed?

Training

When did you undertake your training?

To what extent do you feel that it has equipped you for the nursing tasks that you are required to undertake with patients?

Did you receive instruction in making relationships with patients/ listening/dealing with aggression/control and restraint?

To what extent do you have the opportunity to undertake further training to update your skills?

Have you undertaken any in the last 5 years or so?
If so, what?
If not, why?

What skills do you use in your work?

Do you have any specialist skills that you use with the patient?
If so, what are these?
(Probe: For example, bereavement counselling)

Did you obtain this/these as part of your initial training, or have you acquired them since?

Have there been any significant changes in nursing practice in recent years?

If so, what are they?
What impact has this had on your work?

To what extent are you involved in the assessment/teaching of students/juniors?

What does this involve?

Questions for the qualified named nurse

Admission process

By whom was the patient referred?
What has been the purpose of hospitalisation for the patient?
(Probe: Provision of a safe environment; management of illness)

Were you involved in this process?

If so, what was your role?

Who else was involved?

What was their role?

Whose decision was it to admit the patient?
(Probe: Doctor; nurse and doctor; team decision)

What were the principal criteria used to determine whether to admit the patient?

Is the patient on a section?
If so, is he/she treated differently to other patients?
If so, how?

Assessment process

What are the main purposes of this with respect to the patient?
(Probe: Determination of level of observation; developing a care plan)

What is your role in the process?

Who else is involved?

What is their role?
(Probe: Involvement of relatives; negotiation with patient)

What is the end result of this process?
(Probe: Development of a care plan)
If the patient is on a section ask:

Is the patient treated any differently because he/she is on a section?
If so, how?
(Probe: Observation level)

Inpatient care

How was the patient allocated to the nurse?
(Probe: Named nurse – purpose; advantages/disadvantages)

Did the patient have any choice regarding the named nurse?
(Probe: Sex of named nurse)

Once the person has been admitted and assessed, what specific tasks do you undertake with the patient?

What is/are the purpose of this/these?
(Probe: Seek clarification on: talking to patient – especially if this is linked to therapy/counselling role of nurse; content of conversation; developing a relationship; how long these conversations last; how often you spend time with patients each week; administering medication, dealing with side-effects and reporting back to the doctor; helping with ECT; tending to patients' physical care needs; escorting patients off the ward; observing patients (what do you do when observing those on level 1 and 2 observation?); group sessions involving patient; recreation with patient; skills teaching/treatment advice/relaxation sessions)

To what extent is the patient involved in decisions affecting his/her care?

What kinds of area is the patient involved in?

What is the patient's input into reports on his/her condition at the ward round?
Examples.

What are the principal objectives of the care that you provide to the patient?

To what extent are these objectives reviewed and monitored regarding their continued appropriateness?

How do you determine whether the nursing interventions provided have been successful or not?

Have you been successful with this patient?
Are there written standards of care?
If so, what do they specify?

How much time do you actually spend with the patient?

How is the remainder of your time spent?

What paperwork is associated with patient care?

What other paperwork/office work is there?

How much time does this take on an average shift?

To what extent does this prevent you spending more time with the patient?

Do you work on the night shift?

If so, are there any differences compared with working on day shifts in dealing with the patient?
(Probe: Time with patient)

Working with others

Who else is involved with the patient?

What do they do?
(Probe: Solicitors/meetings – re-detained patients, e.g. appeals)

Whose role is it to ensure that the patient receives the prescribed interventions?
(Probe: Co-ordination of patient care interventions; role of named nurse)

To what extent are there multidisciplinary meetings to discuss the patient's care?

What is the purpose of these?
Is the patient usually involved?
If so, why?
If not, why?

How do your nursing notes relate to the patient's medical notes?

To what extent do you meet with the doctor to discuss the patient's care?

What is the purpose of such meetings?

Is the patient usually involved?
If so, why?
If not, why?

To what extent do you meet with other professionals to discuss the patient's care?

Who else is involved?

What is the purpose of such meetings?

Is the patient usually present?
If so, why?
If not, why?
(Probe: Housing department personnel; DSS personnel about benefits)

To what extent have you discussed the patient's condition with relatives?

To what extent is/are any of the nursing interventions under the clinical supervision of someone else?
If so, who?

What are the interventions involved?

What is the purpose of such supervision?

Discharge process

How do you determine when the patient is ready for discharge?

Whose decision is it?
(Probe: Doctor; multidisciplinary team; patient; community team; hospital team)

What is your role in the process?

Who else is involved?

What is their role?

What is/are the aim/aims of this process for the patient?

Has CPA been offered to any of your patients?

Has this approach been used with any of your patients?

Who was appointed key worker?

Have you had any feedback from the patient or key workers about it?

Whose responsibility is it to ensure that the discharge arrangements are undertaken?
(Probe: A particular individual; a team – hospital and/or community)

How are the hospital and community services co-ordinated?

Do you have networks in the community?

If so, what are they?
How do they link with the hospital?

Whose responsibility is it to ensure that the patient receives the appropriate community care?

To what extent will you be involved with the patient after he/she leaves hospital?

To what extent is this responsibility passed on to someone else?
If so, who?

How is this process managed?

Training

When did you undertake your training?

To what extent do you feel that it has equipped you for the nursing tasks that you are required to undertake with the patient?

Did you receive instruction in making relationships with patients/listening/dealing with aggression/control and restraint?

To what extent do you have the opportunity to undertake further training to update your skills?

Have you undertaken any in the past 5 years or so?
If so, what?
If not, why?

What skills do you use in your work?

Do you have any specialist skills that you use with the patient?
If so, what are these?
(Probe: For example, bereavement counselling)

Did you obtain this/these as part of your initial training, or have you acquired them since?

Have there been any significant changes in nursing practice in recent years?
If so, what are they?

What impact has this had on your work?

To what extent are you involved in the assessment/teaching of students/juniors?

What does this involve?

Questions for unqualified nurses

Admission process

Are you involved in the admission process?
If so, what is your role in the process?

Are you required to do any paperwork?
If so, what is involved?

Are patients on a section treated differently?
If so, in what ways?

To what extent have the types of patient on the ward changed in recent years?
(Probe: Increased 'violence' on the ward; increase in the length of inpatient stay; increase in referrals from police; homelessness; breakdown in community support systems)

Assessment process

Are you involved in the assessment process?

If so, what is your role in the process?
Are you required to do any paperwork?
If so, what is involved?

To what extent are those patients on a section treated differently?
(Probe: Observation level)

Inpatient care

Once a person has been admitted and assessed, what specific tasks do you undertake with the patient?

What is/are the purpose of this/these?
(Probe: Seek clarification on: talking to the patient – especially if this is linked to therapy/counselling role of nurse; content of conversation; developing a relationship; how long these conversations last; how often you spend time with patients each week; administering medication, dealing with side-effects and reporting back to the doctor; helping with ECT; tending to patients' physical care needs; escorting patients off the ward; observing patients (what do you do when observing those on level 1 and 2 observation?) group sessions involving patient; recreation with patient; skills teaching/treatment advice/relaxation sessions)

How much time do you actually spend with patients?

How is the remainder of your time spent?

Are you required to undertake any paperwork/office work?
If so, what is involved?

How much time does this take during an average shift?

To what extent does this prevent you spending more time with patients?

Do you work nights?
If so, are there any differences between the night and day shifts?

What are they?
(Probe: Time with patients)

Have there been any significant changes introduced to do with patient care in the past 5 years or so?
If so, what are they?

Have they affected the care that you provide for the patient?

Working with others

To what extent do you meet with the doctor to discuss the patients' care?

What is the purpose of such meetings?

Is the patient usually involved?
If so, why?
If not, why?

To what extent do you meet with other professionals to discuss the patients' care?

Who else is involved?

What is the purpose of such meetings?

Is the patient usually present?
If so, why?
If not, why?
(Probe: Housing department personnel; DSS personnel about benefits)

To what extent do you meet with relatives to discuss patients' care?

To what extent is/are any of the nursing interventions under the clinical supervision of someone else?
If so, who?

What are the interventions involved?

What is the purpose of such supervision?

Is such practice common?
If so, how long has it been operating?

Discharge process

Are you involved in the discharge process?
If so, what is your role in the process?

Are you required to do any paperwork?
If so, what is involved?

To what extent will you be involved with the patient after he/she leaves hospital?

To what extent is this responsibility passed on to someone else?
If so, who?

How is this process managed?

Training

To what extent do you have the opportunity to undertake further training to update your skills?

Have you undertaken any in the past 5 years or so?
If so, what? If not, why?

What skills do you use in your work?

Do you have any 'specialist' skills that you use with the patient?
If so, what are these?
(Probe: For example, bereavement counselling)

Have there been any significant changes in nursing practice in recent years?

If so, what are they?

What impact have they had on your work?

Questions for patients

Admission

Who arranged for you to come in here?
Why?

Who did you see when you were admitted?

What happens when you are admitted?

Have you been in here before and/or somewhere else?
If so, what was that for?

What did you hope to gain from being in hospital?

Are you getting what you hoped for?

How do you find the ward environment?

In what ways is it beneficial?

Are there any problems with it?
If so, what?

Is the location of the ward within the hospital significant?
If so, how?

Inpatient care

What do you do during the day?

Do you have any treatment off the ward?
If so, by whom and how often?

Do you have any treatment on the ward?
If so, by whom and how often?

What is/are the purpose of this/these?

Do you spend much time talking with other patients?
If so, what do you talk about?

Is there a nurse who is primarily responsible for your care?
If so, who is it?
(Probe: Named nurse)

How often do you see him/her?

How does he/she care for you?

What kind of help do nurses give you?

What is/are the purpose of this/these?

(Probe: Seek clarification on: talking to nurse – especially if this is linked to therapy/counselling role of nurse; content of conversation; developing a relationship; how long these conversations last; how often you spend time with nurses each week; whether this is sufficient; administering medication and dealing with side-effects; attending other treatment on/off the ward; what observation means; group sessions involving nurses; recreation with nurses; skills teaching/treatment advice/relaxation sessions)

Has the help that nurses have given you changed as you have got better?
If so, were you asked about these changes?

Are you getting the care that you feel you need?

Who makes sure that you receive the care that has been prescribed for you?
(Probe: Co-ordination of patient care interventions; role of named nurse)

To what extent would you say that you have been helped by what the nurses have done for you?

How have you been helped?

To what extent have you been involved in decisions affecting your care, such as planning your care with a nurse and agreeing a timetable for receiving particular kinds of help?

What kinds of area are you involved in?

Have there been any benefits and/or problems of such involvement?
If so, what are they?

How much time do you spend with nurses during the day?

What are nurses doing when they are not with patients?

Are there any differences between the day and night?

Is it easier to get hold of a nurse to talk to at night?
Why/why not?

How much time do you spend talking to nurses on duty at night?

And nurses on duty during the day?

If the patient has been in hospital before, ask:

To what extent have you noticed any significant changes in the care that you have received in the past 5 years or so?
If so, what are they?

How have they affected the care that you have received?

Involvement of others

Who else is involved in your care?
(Probe: OT staff; day hospital staff, etc.)

What do you do with them?

To what extent has their involvement helped your recovery?
In what ways?

To what extent are you involved in meetings to discuss your care?

What are they for?

Who is involved?

How do you find these meetings?

To what extent do you meet with a doctor to discuss your care?

When does this happen?

What is the purpose of these meetings?

How do you find these meetings?

To what extent do you meet with other professionals to discuss your care?
If so, who with?
(Probe: Solicitors/CPNs/social workers/psychologists/counsellors)

What is the purpose of such meetings?

How do you find these meetings?

Discharge process

Have you begun to think about leaving the hospital?
If so, was this your idea?

Who else is involved?
(Probe: Housing department personnel and CPNs – personnel with links in the community)

Have you heard of the care programme approach?

Do you know what is meant by it?

Are you/have you used it?

If been in hospital before ask:

Was this approach used when you were last discharged?
If so, how did it work?

How does this approach differ from your experiences of earlier discharges (or how do you expect it to differ)?

Is it better or worse?
Why?

What community support did you receive in the past?

Did this address all your needs?
If not, what unmet needs did you have?

What support do you hope to receive in the future?

Who has been making the arrangements for you to leave hospital?

Is anyone else involved?

To what extent will you have any contact with the hospital once you leave?

Appendix 7
Glossary for nurse and patient schedules

1. **Admission** Activities associated with entry into the service for assessment, treatment or care.

2. **Care planning** (must include patient) Negotiation of care objectives, nursing interventions and time scales between a patient and members of the care team. This is an activity that includes monitoring of achievements, adjustment of care plan and evaluation of outcomes.

3. **Discharge procedure** Activities associated with the actual process of being discharged, such as packing clothes and obtaining discharge information.

4. **Discuss condition with nurse (patient)** Discussion of emotions, feelings and the way in which the condition is experienced by the patient.

5. **Discuss practicalities with nurse (patient)** Discussions related to practical matters such as attendance at occupational therapy, plans for future discharge or facilities available in the community.

6. **Ward round** Meetings of the whole or part of the multidisciplinary care team, with the doctor present, to discuss individual patients. Patients may or may not be seen during the round.

7. **Meeting with doctor** Meeting between doctor and patient to discuss condition, treatment, prognosis or any aspect of present or future care, excluding ward round consultation.

8. **Meeting with other professionals** Meeting between any health or social care professional and patient to discuss condition, treatment, prognosis or any aspect of present or future care. A nurse may or may not be present.

9. **Group sessions on ward** Discussion between a group of patients with similar problems and ward-based staff, e.g. for phobic conditions.

10. **Escort off ward** Nurse supervised movement between ward and another place, where the intention is purely supervisory or protective (*excluding* ECT).

11. **Recreation with nurse (patient)** Any activity jointly undertaken between patient and nurse that would normally be regarded as recreational, such as playing cards or board games, doing jigsaws or any sport.

12. **Outing with nurse (patient)** Any outside walk or outing of a recreational nature by a nurse and patient together, with or without other patients. This would include shopping or visiting places of interest, the country or seaside.

13. **Skills teaching (skills acquisition)** A nurse teaching a patient any skills necessary for self-care. This would include personal hygiene, laundry and cookery lessons.

14. **Treatment advice** Any teaching given by a nurse to a specific patient on that patient's treatment, such as information about prescribed drugs, their self-administration and side-effects.

15. **ECT** Any activity associated with the administration of ECT, to include transfer to the ECT suite through to the recovery process.

16. **Medication** Prescribed medication being administered to individual patients when needed, or administered routinely to one or more patients at the identified time.

17. **Vital signs** Measuring and recording blood pressure, pulse or respiratory rate and volume, or any combination, for individual or groups of patients.

18. **Discussion with relatives** Discussion between nurse and relatives or significant others of the patient's needs, wants, care, treatment and aftercare. The patient may or may not be present. This includes nurses obtaining information for the care plan.

19. **Group recreation** Any recreational activity involving nursing staff and more than one patient (*excluding* watching TV).

20. **Ward meeting** Meeting of ward-based staff and patients to discuss house-keeping issues.

21. **Watching TV** Patient watching TV alone or with other patient and/or a nurse.

22. **Assistance with personal care** Personal care activities such as dressing, washing, cooking or eating, with the assistance of a nurse.

PATIENT SCHEDULE ONLY

23. **Treatment off the ward** Attending treatment sessions off ward (*excluding* ECT), such as occupational therapy, without the supervision of a nurse.

24. **Ward tasks** Undertaking any tasks that would be described as house-keeping, such as washing dishes, or hospitality, such as making and handing out tea to others.

25. **Visitors** Any activity with visitors. It may be off the ward, e.g. having tea in the cafe. *Does not* include discussion between relatives and a nurse about patient's condition.

26. **Talk with patient (condition)** Talking with fellow patients about condition, personal feelings and life experiences.

27. **Recreation without nurse** Activity normally regarded as recreational that *does not* involve nursing staff. This includes 'chatting' to other patients and ancillary staff.

28. **Outing without nurse** Any outside walk or outing of a recreational nature, alone or with other patients, but *not* accompanied by a nurse. This would include shopping or visiting places of interest.

29. **Home on trial** A period of time off the ward in their own home or elsewhere, e.g. a rehabilitation centre.

30. **Self-care** Activities considered to be self-care, such as dressing, washing, cooking or eating without the supervision or direct involvement of a member of staff.

31. **Doing nothing** Sitting, standing, walking or lying down without obvious purpose. This would include sleeping during the day.

32. **Asleep during the night** This relates to sleep after official 'lights-out'.

33. **Not asleep during the night** This relates to periods when the patient is not asleep after the official 'lights-out'.

34. **Other**.

NURSE SCHEDULE ONLY

23. **Assessment** Observing, recording, analysing and interpreting the patients' physical appearance, social behaviour and apparent psychological and emotional status for input into care plans and for monitoring and evaluation of outcomes.

24. **Hand-over** One nurse handing over to another nurse responsibility for one or more patients.

25. **Ward management** Any task related to ward management, e.g. checking staff cover.

26. **Close observation** Observation and assessment of the patient by a nurse, either within touching distance of the patient or keeping the patient within sight at all times.

27. **General observation** Observing more than one patient and checking the environment.

28. **Crisis intervention** Dealing with unexpected, unplanned events.

29. **Teaching/assessing students** Activities intended to assess or improve the professional skills or knowledge of students and juniors, and the associated paperwork.

30. **Patients' notes** Reading or recording data in patients' nursing or medical records, including updating care plans.

31. **Clerical/telephone** General clerical or telephone duties such as ordering stock or booking ambulances.

32. **Errands** Activities that take the nurse off the ward, such as collecting from the pharmacy or the delivery of specimens.

33. **Breaks** Official coffee, lunch or tea breaks.

34. **Interpersonal** Activities that are not work related and not in official break time, such as conversations about private life and activities between staff.

35. **Other**.

Figure A7.1 Patient activity schedule

Hospital: Ward: Shift: Date: Hour:

Patient's name

	00	15	30	45	00	15	30	45	00	15	30	45	00	15	30	45	00	15	30	45
1. Admission																				
2. Care planning (discuss with nurse)																				
3. Discharge procedure																				
4. Discuss condition with nurse																				
5. Discuss practicalities with nurse																				
6. Ward round																				
7. Meeting with doctor																				
8. Meeting with other professionals																				
9. Group sessions on ward																				
10. Escort off ward																				
11. Recreation with nurse																				
12. Outing with nurse																				
13. Skills acquisition																				
14. Treatment advice																				
15. ECT																				
16. Medication																				
17. Vital signs																				
18. Discussion with relatives																				
19. Group recreation																				
20. Ward meeting																				
21. Watching TV																				

(contd)

Figure A7.1 (contd)

Hospital: Ward: Shift: Date: Hour:

Patient's name

	00	15	30	45	00	15	30	45	00	15	30	45	00	15	30	45
22. Assistance with personal care																
23. Treatment off ward																
24. Ward tasks																
25. Visitors																
26. Talk with patient (condition)																
27. Recreation without nurse																
28. Outing without nurse																
29. Home on trial																
30. Self-care																
31. Doing nothing																
32. Asleep during the night																
33. Not asleep during the night																
34. Other																

Figure A7.2 Nurse activity list

Hospital: Ward: Shift: Date: Hour:

Nurse's name

	00	15	30	45	00	15	30	45	00	15	30	45	00	15	30	45
1. Admission																
2. Care planning (must include patient)																
3. Discharge procedure																
4. Discuss condition with patient																
5. Discuss practicalities with patient																
6. Ward round																
7. Meeting with doctor																
8. Meeting with other professionals																
9. Group sessions on ward																
10. Escort off ward																
11. Recreation with patient																
12. Outing with patient																
13. Skills teaching																
14. Treatment advice																
15. ECT																
16. Medication																
17. Vital signs																
18. Discussion with relatives																
19. Group recreation																
20. Ward meeting																
21. Watching TV																

(contd)

Figure A7.2 (contd)

Hospital: Ward: Shift: Date: Hour:

Nurse's name

	00	15	30	45	00	15	30	45	00	15	30	45	00	15	30	45
22. Assistance with personal care																
23. Assessment																
24. Hand-over																
25. Ward management																
26. Close observation																
27. General observation																
28. Crisis intervention																
29. Teaching/assessing students																
30. Patient's notes																
31. Clerical/telephone																
32. Errands																
33. Breaks																
34. Interpersonal																
35. Other																

Appendix 8
Report on the qualitative pre-pilot project

1. Introduction

1.1 This report presents the principal findings that have emerged during the qualitative pre-pilot work undertaken in Bootham Park Hospital, York and the General Infirmary, Pontefract.

2. Nurse interviews

2.1 In total, two group interviews (one per site) and six individual interviews (four in York and two in Pontefract) were undertaken.

2.2 The following is a summary of the principal nursing tasks identified during the interviews:

1. The admission and assessment procedures.

2. Providing a safe and ordered environment, including giving patients the appropriate level of observation. Moreover, to 'stabilise' the patient – in conjunction with medication – to ensure that patients are not a risk to themselves or to others.

3. Administering medication prescribed by doctors and reporting to them any adverse effects on patients.

4. Dealing with 'crises' such as violent outbursts by patients.

5. Preparation for, and aiding recovery from, ECT.

6. Attending to patients' physical care needs.

7. Escorting patients off the ward, both within and outside the hospital.

8. Liaising with other agencies/professionals.

9. Responding to patients' requests to discuss practical matters, for example in relation to their discharge.

10. Responding to patients' requests to discuss how they feel or initiating a discussion with a patient to 'open up' (if they have sufficient time).

11. Dealing with the paperwork associated with students or patient care, for example updating a care plan.

12. Supervising students.

2.3 A number of other issues were also identified:

Referrals
These usually, but not exclusively, come from GPs. Referrals are also received from a variety of other sources, including CPNs, social workers, outpatient departments, day hospital staff and 'self-referrals'.

Admittance
A doctor is informed of the new arrival. The doctor will then perform a thorough physical examination, and the patient is interviewed to compile a brief life history on, for example, why they are there, whether they are taking any medication, whether they have received psychiatric help in the past, and so on.

Assessment

1. For the first 72 hours, an 'informal' assessment of the patient's condition is undertaken. The principal aims are to decide the appropriate 'observation level' (or 'obs') for the patient, to determine the interventions required and to begin to identify the psychiatric problems. There are four 'obs' levels:

- A obs: rare, usually reserved for someone on a 'section'. The patient must be within touching distance of a nurse.

- B obs: a nurse must be able to see the patient at all times.

- C obs: the whereabouts of the patient must be known at all times. The patient can leave the ward, but *with* a nurse escort.

- D obs: as for C, but *without* a nurse escort.

Most people are on level 'C' or 'D' obs.

2. A formal *care plan* must be prepared by the end of 72 hours (although, on one ward in Pontefract, which had a number of elderly patients, 7 days were allowed before the preparation of the plan).

Care Plan

This consists of:

1. A statement of the problem(s)/issue(s).

2. A list of the 'interventions' needed, including physical needs, medical needs and 'mental' needs.

3. It specifies the *named nurse* (seen as the patient's 'advocate').

4. Review dates for particular issues to ensure its continued appropriateness.

Discharge

1. This is co-ordinated by the 'named nurse'. A multidiscipli-nary team (MDT) is generally convened to discuss commu-nity support. The patient is usually present.

2. The *'care programme approach'* is usually used for those with 'complex needs' and/or who require numerous service inputs. For a 'simple' problem, it would suffice to inform the GP.

Therapeutic role

1. This consists largely of *talking to and listening to* the patient in the 'calm and relaxed environment' of the hospital ward. This is perceived as a central component of a patient's treatment. (Some nurses referred to this as 'counselling'.) One of the objectives of this is to encourage confidence-building and the development of a trusting relationship with the patient. It also allows the patient to acknowledge and to begin to address his or her problem(s).

2. Patients are 'encouraged' to participate in some form of 'programme' – particularly in York – usually occupational therapy. This helps to provide a structure to the day and prevents patients from dwelling, 'negatively', on their problems. This is seen as therapy/rehabilitation.

3. 'Formal' therapies, for example bereavement counselling and occupational therapy, are undertaken by others off the ward. Few nurses have 'specialist' skills to undertake such work.

4. ECT is used, but for small numbers of patients at any one time. Its main purpose is to lift depression.

Role of doctors
Medical staff appear to have little direct day-to-day involvement with patients. The principal involvement of doctors is when patients are first admitted and during ward rounds. Doctors tend to respond to reports made to them by nurses and/or other staff such as, occupational therapists, rather than directly by patients. Nurses report on such matters as the effect of medication on patients.

Other agencies

1. If patients do not respond to the care provided in the acute setting, they will be referred somewhere else, for example a long-stay ward or a local authority residential home.

2. Local authorities do not deal with acutely ill patients. This is always done in a hospital. The role of local authorities is in the provision of residential care and day care.

3. Patient interviews

3.1 In total, 11 patients were interviewed – 6 in York and 5 in Pontefract.

3.2 The principle issues identified during the interviews were as follows.

Role of nurses

1. Nurses tend to 'encourage' patients to go to occupational therapy (particularly in York). This was for 'therapeutic' reasons.

2. Once admitted, patients said that they had little contact with nurses. Nurses did, however, make time to see patients if requested. A lot of nursing time was taken up with 'obs' and 'sitting in the office doing paperwork'.

3. All patients knew what a 'named' nurse/key worker was and could name their own.

4. The principal tasks that nurses perform with patients are:

    •   To make sure their *physical needs* are addressed, for example that medication is taken.
    •   To take the '*pressure off*' patients and to provide a safe environment. (All patients liked the nurses caring for them.)
    •   They help to provide a *structured day*, for example patients are encouraged to go to occupational therapy (particularly in York).
    •   To prepare them to *cope* in the 'outside world'.
    •   To sort out *discharge arrangements.*

Benefits of being in hospital

1. Most patients mentioned the benefits of talking about their problems to other patients. (They appeared to talk more to each other than to the nurses!)

2. The hospital provided a secure and safe environment. It gave patients the 'space' to 'think things through'. It also allowed them opportunities to talk to professionals who were experienced in dealing with mental health problems.

3. 'Doing something' during the day was seen as important by most patients. It helped to 'take their mind off' their problems. Most patients tried to get off the ward if they could, even if it was only for a walk.

4. Most patients found that the evenings/weekends were the worst times – 'there is nothing to do'.

Therapy

1. Most 'formal' therapies/treatment happened off the ward. (In Pontefract, many of the services, for example psychotherapy and the day hospital, were located on site. These services were also available to outpatients.)

2. ECT was seen as beneficial in helping to alleviate depression.

Role of doctors
Once admitted, patients saw little of the doctors. They generally only saw them for a few minutes each week on ward rounds.

User choice and involvement

1. Overall, there was little choice about what patients could do and when (this contrasting with what nurses said). Their lives in hospital were highly 'routinised'. (This was mentioned particularly by patients in Pontefract. This could have been due to the fact that there were often only 3/4 nurses on duty on a 28-bed ward. This was in contrast to York, where 3/4 nurses were often on duty, but on wards of 15–20 beds.)

2. A number of patients said that they had some input into the development of their own care plan. Both sites had 'community meetings' (ward meetings where patients could raise issues about the running of the ward but *not* individual problems).

3. Most patients said that they were given little information by nurses/doctors about 'the system'. Most patients 'picked things up' from other patients.

4. Conclusion

4.1 The main conclusions to be drawn from this analysis of qualitative pre-pilot work are that:

1. Nurses appeared to have only small therapeutic role. The main functions were 'custodial' and administrative.

2. The main benefit for patients was the opportunity to be 'removed' from their everyday existence and to begin to address their problems in a safe and relaxed environment.

INTERVIEW TOPICS FOR THE NURSE AND PATIENT INTERVIEWS

Introduction

This paper provides an indication of the principal areas to be covered during the interviews with nurses and patients. The interviews will relate to specific patients.

Nurses

1. *Admission*
    • role and purpose
    • role and purpose of nurse
    • involvement of others, including doctors.

2. *Assessment*
    • role and purpose
    • role and purpose of nurse
    • development of care plan
    • involvement of others, including doctors.

3. *Time in hospital*
    • role and purpose: providing a 'safe environment', 'stabilising' the patient's condition
    • role and purpose of nursing care
    • administering medication and dealing with side-effects
    • dealing with 'crises'
    • helping with ECT
    • tending to patients' physical care needs
    • escorting patients off the ward

- talking to patients about their care
- involvement of patients in their care
- paperwork, including supervising students
- observing patients
- therapeutic role
- liaison with other hospital staff/departments, including occupational therapists
- ward meetings with/without patients
- role of the 'named nurse'
- training for nursing, including specialists in, for example, bereavement counselling.

4. *Discharge*
   - role and purpose
   - role and purpose of nurse
   - 'care programme approach'
   - involvement of others
   - liaison with community agencies/professionals
   - determining when patients are ready for discharge

Patients

- daily routines
- identify 'named nurse'
- their needs by day/night
- whether their needs are met
- involvement in decisions affecting their treatment
- role and purpose of nurses
- views on nursing care provided
- expectations about purpose of hospitalisation
- how conductive is the environment to their recovery?

Appendix 9
Report on the qualitative pilot project

1. Executive summary

1.1 The pilot was undertaken successfully in one location. The staff on the ward concerned were extremely helpful and co-operative throughout the fieldwork period.

1.2 During the pilot, the researchers were able to test fieldwork procedures and research instruments, and to develop a method to analyse transcript material.

1.3 The researchers were able to obtain all the required data. However, difficulties were experienced by the Information Officer in obtaining data on past patients following the recent establishment of the Wakefield and Pontefract Community Health Trust.

1.4 Minor amendments were made to researchers' procedures and research instruments, including restructuring the nurse interview questions.

1.5 Feedback from ward staff was positive, and nurses' comments assisted researchers in making additional amendments to their procedures and research instruments.

1.6 The researchers were able to use the relevant data to prepare district, hospital and ward profiles.

1.7 Material from nurse and patient interviews, observational data and material collected during ward rounds and hand-overs were used to describe the activities performed by mental health nurses, and to identify the perceptions of psychiatric patients of their care.

2. Introduction

2.1 The purpose of the pilot was threefold:

1. to test the fieldwork procedures;
2. to test the research instruments;
3. to devise a method for analysing the interview transcripts.

2.2 The fieldwork was undertaken as planned. Details are described in section 3 below.

2.3 During the week before the pilot took place, the researchers met with the mental health manager and the ward manager to discuss practical arrangements. Both managers were given *pro formas* to complete, and the ward manager was interviewed. It was agreed to meet with them on the last day of the fieldwork to discuss the experience of the pilot.

2.4 The pilot was undertaken on one ward at Pontefract General Infirmary from 28 February to 4 March 1994.

2.5 The staff were extremely helpful to the researchers throughout the fieldwork, and positive relationships were established with them.

3. The pilot

3.1 During the pilot, all data sought were successfully obtained.

3.2 Staff duty lists were recorded on the first day of the fieldwork, and any subsequent amendments were recorded on the last day of the fieldwork.

3.3 Interviews took place with 11 day and 2 night nurses. The grades of the day staff were as follows: one F, two E, three D and five A. The grades of the night staff were F and E. Additional information on the work undertaken at night was obtained during interviews with auxiliaries on day duty who rotated to nights.

3.4 Data were provided by the ward manager on staffing levels during December 1998 and during February 1994.

3.5 A list of patients on the ward was recorded on the first day of the fieldwork, and any subsequent amendments were recorded on the last day of the fieldwork. Certain data were added to the ward patient list, such as their age, gender, observation level and diagnosis, and whether any of them were detained under the 1983 Mental Health Act.

3.6 Patient dependency data were obtained from the ward manager, and the dependency levels were calculated.

3.7 Patients were randomly selected for interview and observation, and any refusals recorded. The characteristics of patients who refused to participate were compared with those of all patients on the ward.

3.8 Interviews were conducted with four of the five selected patients; the last patient was unwell on the last day of the fieldwork when her interview was scheduled.

3.9 Data on patients were sought from the Information Officer relating to existing and past patients, such as the number of admissions and discharges, average lengths of stay, location on discharge, and bed complement and occupancy levels. Difficulties were experienced obtaining this information because the psychiatric wards were now part of a different Trust from the rest of the hospital. This new Mental Health Trust did not have past records of ward patients.

3.10 Observation of the nursing staff on duty and of five selected patients took place over three shifts: one night, one early and one late day. Two observers were used as a test of reliability. Subsequently, the two sets of observations were collated and compared. In general, there was broad agreement between the two, and differences were often attributed to observations being taken at different times within the 15-minute observation periods.

3.11 During the course of the fieldwork period, the researchers attended two ward rounds and the hand-overs between the early and late day shifts.

3.12 A feedback session took place on the final day of the fieldwork, which was attended by the mental health manager, the ward manager and the researchers. The ward manager had obtained feedback from his staff, and presented us with written comments.

4.   Lessons from the pilot

4.1   Feedback from ward staff

4.1.1 The feedback from ward staff was positive. They did not find the experience too intimidating, and they reported that interviews were undertaken professionally and sensitively.

4.1.2 The researchers were most grateful for the assistance provided by staff throughout the fieldwork period. They were aware that long interviews with nurses created additional work for their colleagues on duty.

4.1.3 The concern of nurses that observers might not be aware that they may be performing several activities at the same time was noted. The nurse observer will need to ask the nurses when she has any doubts about particular activities.

4.1.4 The concern of nurses about the effect that frequent observations might have on patients was noted. To address this concern, certain procedures have been amended. On the first day of fieldwork, it is proposed that the researchers will attend the ward community meeting to introduce themselves to the patients, to explain their role on the ward and to provide information about the project. When patients agree to participate in the research, it will be brought to their attention that they will be observed during three specific shifts.

4.1.5 The difficulty encountered by nurses with regard to the nurse questionnaire has been recognised. The instrument has been amended to include an additional column to enable nurses to indicate whether activities performed occasionally form part of their regular duties.

4.1.6 The concern of ward nurses about patient confidentiality, particularly during hand-overs, was noted. The researchers had stressed the confidential nature of all the material collected during the study in their discussions with the mental health manager and the ward manager. These managers had made clear to ward staff that they were satisfied with the researchers' assurances regarding confidentiality.

4.2   Modifications to research instruments

4.2.1 The researchers identified the benefit of having five sets of questions for nurses to cover the following categories of nurses:

- qualified nursing staff at night;
- unqualified nursing staff at night;
- unqualified day staff;
- qualified key workers of selected patients;
- qualified staff who were not key workers of selected patients.

4.2.2 The researchers identified some additional questions to ask both the patients and the nurses. Additional questions to add to the patients' list were as follows:

- interactions with other patients;
- their experiences of the admission process;
- the availability of nurses to talk to them at night.

Additional questions to add to the nurses' list were as follows:

- sectioning;
- work involving solicitors.

4.2.3 Additional questions have been added to the interview schedule with ward managers:

- timing of occupational and other therapy sessions;
- nurses' breaks and mealtimes;
- times when nurses are not available for interviews;
- whether students would be on the ward during the fieldwork.

4.2.4 Additional diagnoses and sections under the 1983 Mental Health Act have been added to relevant *pro formas* (ward patient and ward manager *pro formas*).

4.2.5 Certain *pro formas* (ward environment, patient and staff lists) have been modified for easier usage.

4.2.6 Minor changes have been made to the nurse and patient observation lists and the glossary.

4.3   *Procedural changes*

4.3.1 The list of topics to be covered during the initial visit to the site has been extended to include the following:

- availability of car parking;
- times when food is available during the day and night;
- arrangement for a feedback session.

4.3.2 Both researchers will be present during patient interviews. This will provide the interviewer with assistance should the patient become upset or disturbed during the interview.

4.3.3 The observation of the night shift will take place after the early and late day shifts. This will enable the observer to become familiar with the ward before covering the night shift.

5.   Use of data

5.1 The staff duty list and information on present and past staffing were used in the preparation of staff profile.

5.2 The ward list, dependency data and information on present and past patients were used in the preparation of a profile of ward patients.

5.3 Data from the mental health manager and the ward manager, and the ward environment data, were used in the preparation of district, hospital and ward profiles.

5.4 Data from ward rounds and hand-over sessions were used to feed into the analyses of patient and nurse transcript material (see section 6.5 below). They were also used to provide information on the following:

- the use that was made of nursing care plans;
- who was present, and how these meetings were conducted;
- what arrangements were made for inpatients to see other therapists or professionals (e.g. solicitors, housing personnel, social workers or CPNs);
- how discharges were planned, and whether all patients were offered the care programme approach;
- unforeseen events/occurrences, which might otherwise have been missed.

5.5 Observational data were used to feed into the analysis of nurse and patient transcript material (see section 5.6 below).

5.6 From an examination of the data, *pro formas* were developed for both the nurse transcript material and the patient transcript material. Interview material from the five selected patients and their key workers was compared, as was additional information added from observations of them and from material collected during the ward rounds and hand-overs. Interview material from the remaining nurses was analysed in a similar manner, omitting the comparison with patient transcripts. This 'triangulation' enabled the researchers to comment on the validity of the generalised information.

5.7 The categories used to examine the nurse and patient transcript materials are attached (see below).

6. Conclusions

6.1 The original research questions to be addressed by this study were identified as follows:

- What is the patient population in acute psychiatric settings, and how has this population changed in recent years?

- What is the nursing population in terms of the numbers on duty and the qualifications of nurses?

- What activities are performed by nurses caring for acute psychiatric patients?

- What is the patients' perception of the nurses' role in relation to their needs and expectations?

6.2 The existing literature on the activities performed by nurses caring for acute psychiatric patients concentrates on nurse–patient interactions, and the literature on the skills of mental health nurses concentrates on communication and 'counselling' skills. Numerous studies have shown, however, that nurse–patient interactions occur infrequently and last for only a short period of time.

6.3 This study utilises some of the methods used in earlier studies such as observing nurse activities and using semi-structured interview techniques. It aims to provide evidence from 12 sites on the amount of time nurses spend with patients, and how that time is spent during a 1-week period. Nurses will also be questioned about the extent to which their training prepared them for the work required of them.

6.4 The literature fails to explore how mental health nurses spend their time when they are not interacting with patients. This study explores that issue.

6.5 The literature on the perceptions of psychiatric patients of their care is limited. This study explores patient perceptions through interviews and compares and contrasts views expressed by patients with observations of the activities of those patients, and the nurses on duty, during three shifts in each location.

6.6 The pilot has shown that the research approach adopted will enable the research questions listed above to be addressed.

Feedback from staff

Prior to the research being carried out, based on the information conveyed to staff, there was an expectancy that the experience would be very intimidating. This was not found to be the case. Staff reported that the interviews were carried out very professionally and sensitively and that they did not feel threatened or intimidated.

The presence of the researchers had an obvious disruption on the activities of the nurses. Colleagues were missing for long periods of time.

Nurses made an analogy between being observed at 15-minute intervals and patients being put on level 3 observations; this was very enlightening and gave the nurses more insight into the effects they have on patients who are under close observation.

The nurses, while being observed, questioned whether the observers understood the reason why they were doing certain things and whether they recognised that while doing one particular activity, they might in fact be performing several activities at the same time.

Some nurses were worried about the effect that the frequent observation was having on the patients who were not on close observation as planned by the nurse, although this had been discussed with the patients during community meetings.

The questionnaires asked for certain information but the nurses felt frustrated that some information that they would like to have put across was not included in the structure of the questionnaire.

Some disappointment was expressed that one afternoon several situations arose that involved crisis counselling sessions, and also group relaxation took place, but there was no observer around for this span of duty.

There was some concern about patient confidentiality, especially during the hand-over period when sensitive issues were being discussed.

Pro formas for analysing transcripts

Categories for qualified nursing staff (day and night)

Involvement with patients
- close observations of individual patients
- general observation of patients
- talking to patients – 'social'
- talking to patients – conditions/practicalities
- assisting with personal care
- escorting
- differences between sectioned/non-sectioned patients
- recreation
- community ward meeting
- admissions
- assessment
- care plan
- care programme approach
- allocation to named nurse

Treatment
- drugs
- ECT
- therapy
- other

Supervising untrained nursing staff

Involvement with other professionals
- hospital
- community

- clinical supervision

Involvement with students
- assessing
- mentoring

Involvement with relatives

General ward tasks
- housekeeping – cleaning/tidying
- observations of ward environment
- ward meetings of staff (patients not present)
- clerical – general
- clerical – patients
- errands
- ward management
- ward rounds – use of care plans; role of nurse; how conducted
- hand-over – use of care plans; how conducted

Dealing with unexpected ward events

Training

Specialist skills

Changes
- ward
- nursing

Other

Categories for unqualified nursing staff (day and night)

Involvement with patients
- close observation of individual patients
- general observation of patients
- talking to patients – 'social'
- talking to patients – condition/practicalities
- assisting with personal care
- escorting
- differences between sectioned/non-sectioned patients
- recreation
- community ward meetings

Assisting qualified nursing staff
- admissions
- assessment
- discharge
- treatments

Involvement with other professionals
- hospital
- community

Involvement with relatives

General ward tasks
- housekeeping – cleaning/tidying
- observations of ward environment
- ward meetings of staff (patients not present)
- clerical – general
- clerical – patients
- errands

Dealing with unexpected ward events

Training

Specialist skills

Changes
- ward
- nursing

Other

Categories of patient

Involvement with other patients
- talking – 'social'
- talking – condition

Involvement with nurses
- talking – 'social'
- talking – condition

- care planning
- care programme approach
- recreation

Treatment
- drugs
- ECT
- therapy
- other

Involvement with other professionals
- hospital
- community

Involvement with relatives

General ward tasks
- housekeeping – cleaning/tidying
- community ward meetings
- errands for staff

Life on the ward – day
- location prior to hospitalisation
- purpose of hospitalisation
- benefits of hospitalisation
- problems of hospitalisation
- previous periods of hospitalisation

Life on the ward – night

Other

Appendix 10
Patient profile

Name: Case number:

Hospital:

Date of admission:

Numbers of weeks in hospital:

Readmitted within 2 weeks of discharge:

On an acute psychiatric ward before:

By whom referred:

Location prior to admission:

Anticipated location on discharge, if different from above:

Knows name of key worker or named nurse:

Appendix 11
Nurse activity and personal details questionnaire

Hospital: Ward:

Case number:

Please refer to the attached glossary of terms.

Please tick <u>one</u> of the boxes for each of the activities listed:

Frequent	=	activity performed frequently as part of your regular duties.
Infrequent	=	activity performed infrequently as part of your regular duties
Not normal duty	=	activity that is not one you would normally be expected to carry out
Never	=	activity you are never asked to perform.

	Frequent	Infrequent	Not normal duty	Never
1. Admission				
2. Care planning (must include patient)				
3. Discharge procedure				
4. One-to-one discussion with patient				
5. Doing nothing				
6. Ward round				
7. Meeting with doctor				
8. Meeting with other professionals				
9. Group sessions on ward				
10. Escort off ward				
11. Recreation with patient				
12. Outing with patient				
13. Skills teaching				
14. Treatment advice				
15. ECT				
16. Medication/dressing				
17. Vital signs				
18. Discussion with relatives				
19. Comforting/controlling a patient				
20. Ward meeting				

(contd)

	Frequent	Infrequent	Not normal duty	Never
21. Watching TV				
22. Assistance with personal care				
23. Assessment				
24. Hand-over				
25. Office duties				
26. Close observation				
27. General observation				
28. Crisis intervention				
29. Teaching/assessing students				
30. Liaising with other professionals				
31. Domestic duties				
32. Errands				
33. Breaks during shift				
34. Interpersonal				
35. Other (please specify)				

Please could you provide the following personal details:

Age: Gender: Grade:

Time in service:

Please circle one category from each of the two lists below:

Work: 1.   Full time

             2.   Part time

Work on: 1.   Permanent days

             2.   Permanent nights

             3.   Internal rotation days to night

             4.   Internal rotation nights to days

             5.   Internal rotation equally on days and nights.

Please give details on qualifications, with dates:

RMN

RGN

State Enrolled Nurse (Mental Illness)

State Enrolled Nurse (General)

Degree

Further professional qualifications entered on the UKCC register

Thank you for providing this information.

Glossary of terms

Nurse Schedule

1. **Admission** Activities associated with entry into the service for assessment, treatment or care.

2. **Care planning** (must include patient) Negotiation of care objectives, nursing interventions and time scales between a patient and members of the care team. This is an activity that includes monitoring of achievements, adjustment of care plan and evaluation of outcomes.

3. **Discharge procedure** Activities associated with the actual process of being discharged, such as packing clothes and obtaining discharge information.

4. **One-to-one discussion – nurse and patient** This includes general discussion, practical matters such as attendance at occupational therapy, plans for future discharge or facilities available in the community, and discussion of emotions, feelings and the way the condition is experienced by the patient.

5. **Doing nothing** Nurse or patient sitting, standing or walking around without obvious purpose. This would include the patient lying in bed doing nothing during the day, i.e. 8.00 a.m. until the night shift starts.

6. **Ward round** Meetings of the whole or part of the multidisciplinary care team, with the doctor present, to discuss individual patients. Patients may or may not be seen during the round.

7. **Meeting with the doctor** Meeting between doctor and patient to discuss condition, treatment, prognosis or any aspect of present or future care, excluding ward round consultation.

8. **Meeting with other professionals** Meeting between any health- or social care professional and patient to discuss condition, treatment, prognosis or any aspect of present or future care. It also includes meetings with solicitors, the police, housing department personnel and social security staff. The meeting may take place off the ward, for example in a social worker's office. A nurse may or may not be present.

9. **Group sessions on ward** Discussion between a group of patients with similar problems and ward-based staff, for example for phobic conditions.

10. **Escort off ward** Nurse supervised movement between the ward and another place, where the intention is purely supervisory or protective (*excluding* ECT).

11. **Recreation with nurse (patient)** Any activity jointly undertaken between one or more patients and one or more nurses that would normally be regarded as recreational, such as playing cards and board games, doing jigsaws or any sport. This does not include watching TV.

12. **Outing with nurse (patient)** Any outside walk or outing of a recreational nature by a nurse and patient together, with or without other patients. This would include shopping or visiting places of interest, the country or seaside.

13. **Skills teaching (skills acquisition)** A nurse teaching a patient any skills necessary for self-care. This would include personal hygiene, laundry and cookery lessons.

14. **Treatment advice** Any teaching given by a nurse to a specific patient on that patient's treatment, such as information about prescribed drugs, their self-administration and side-effects.

15. **ECT** Any activity associated with the administration of ECT, to include transfer to the ECT suite through to the recovery process.

16. **Medication** Prescribed medications being administered to individual patients when needed, or administered routinely to one or more patients at the identified time.

17. **Vital signs** Measuring and recording blood pressure, pulse or respiratory rate and volume, or any combination, for individual or groups of patients.

18. **Discussion with relatives** Discussion between nurse and relatives or significant others of the patient's needs, wants, care, treatment and aftercare. The patient may or may not be present. This includes nurses obtaining information for the care plan.

19. **Comforting/controlling a patient** A nurse comforting a distressed patient or controlling an unruly patient (*excluding* watching TV).

20. **Ward meeting** Meetings of ward-based staff and patients to discuss house-keeping issues.

21. **Watching TV** Patient watching TV alone or with other patient and/or a nurse.

22. **Assistance with personal care** Personal care activities such as dressing, washing, cooking or eating, with the assistance of a nurse.

23. **Assessment** Observing, recording, analysing and interpreting the patient's physical appearance, social behaviour and apparent psychological and emotional status for input into care plans and for monitoring and evaluating of outcomes.

24. **Hand-over** One nurse handing over to another nurse responsibility for one or more patients.

25. **Office duties** Reading or recording data in patients' nursing or medical records, including updating care plans.

26. **Close observation** Observation and assessment of the patient by a nurse, either within touching distance of the patient, or keeping the patient within sight at all times.

27. **General observation** Observing more than one patient and checking the environment.

28. **Crisis intervention** Dealing with unexpected, unplanned events.

29. **Teaching/assessing students** Activities intended to assess or improve the professional skills or knowledge of students and juniors, and the associated paperwork.

30. **Liaising with other professionals** Meeting or liaising with other professionals, including solicitors or police, on patient matters in the absence of the patient.

31. **Domestic duties** Tidying or cleaning the ward and dealing with the ward laundry or checking stocks.

32. **Errands** Activities that take the nurse off the ward, such as collecting from the pharmacy or the delivery of specimens.

33. **Breaks during shift** Any period of time, on or off the ward during a shift, when the nurse has a break from his or her duties, such as coffee, lunch or tea breaks. This includes periods spent being interviewed by the researchers.

34. **Interpersonal** Activities that are not work related and not in official break time, such as conversations about private life and activities between staff.

35. **Not known** Unable to ascertain whereabouts of nurse.

Appendix 12
Postal survey of
Trust profiles

To be completed by the Mental Health Manager

Name of NHS Trust: ....

Hospital (or other type of facility): ....

Name and telephone number (to be contact only in case of query):

....

Date : ....

STAFF INFORMATION (for acute mental health services at 31 March 1994)

Hospital mental health staff

1. *Nursing staff:*

	Funded establishment	In post
Grade I	. . .	. . .
Grade H	. . .	. . .
Grade G	. . .	. . .
Grade F	. . .	. . .
Grade E	. . .	. . .
Grade D1	. . .	. . .
Grade D2 (Enrolled Nurse)	. . .	. . .
Grade C	. . .	. . .

Grade B   . . .   . . .
Grade A   . . .   . . .

2. Qualified grades of the following staff

Qualified outreach/link nurses   . . .   . . .
Occupational therapists (total for all grades)   . . .   . . .
Physiotherapists   . . .   . . .
Psychologists   . . .   . . .

3. Medical staff

Consultants   . . .   . . .
Registrars   . . .   . . .
Senior house officers   . . .   . . .

4. Specifically employed counsellors (e.g. family or bereavement counsellors, please specify):

....

....

5. Other (please specify)

....

....

Community mental health staff

	Funded establishment	In post

6. Community nursing staff

	Funded establishment	In post
Grade I	. . .	. . .
Grade H	. . .	. . .
Grade G	. . .	. . .
Grade F	. . .	. . .
Grade E	. . .	. . .
Grade D1	. . .	. . .

Grade D2 (Enrolled Nurse)   . . .   . . .
Grade C   . . .   . . .
Grade B   . . .   . . .
Grade A   . . .   . . .

7. *Qualified grades of the following staff*

Occupational therapists   . . .   . . .
Physiotherapists (total for all grades)   . . .   . . .
Psychologists   . . .   . . .

8. *Medical staff*

Consultants   . . .   . . .
Registrars   . . .   . . .
Senior house officers   . . .   . . .

9. *Specifically employed counsellors* (e.g. family or bereavement counsellors)

....

....

10. *Other* (please specify):

....

....

Hospital facilities (for acute mental health services at 31 March 1994)

11. Number of acute mental health beds   . . .
    within general hospital   (e.g. under 65)
    (If applicable, specify whether age
    criteria apply)   . . .
                                              (e.g. over 65)

12. Number of acute mental health beds
    in private hospitals within the
    boundary of your main purchasing
    authority   . . .

13. Number of acute mental health beds within long-stay (Water Tower) hospitals   . . .

14. Other acute mental health facilities (please specify, with bed numbers)

....

....

....

Community facilities

15. *Inpatient NHS facilities* (for acute psychiatric patients at 31 March 1994)

	Number of beds
Crisis/emergency	. . .
Intensive care	. . .
Personality/behavioural disorders	. . .
Alcohol/drug/substance misuse	. . .

Other (please specify)

....

....

....

16. *Grades of staff working in community inpatient facilities* (at 31 March 1994)

	Funded establishment	In post
Grade I	. . .	. . .
Grade H	. . .	. . .
Grade G	. . .	. . .
Grade F	. . .	. . .
Grade E	. . .	. . .

Grade D1   . . .   . . .
Grade D2 (Enrolled Nurse)   . . .   . . .
Grade C   . . .   . . .
Grade B   . . .   . . .
Grade A   . . .   . . .

17. *Outpatient NHS facilities* (for acute psychiatric patients at 31 March 1994)

Number of mental health day hospitals
(If applicable, specify if age criteria apply)   . . .
                                                 (e.g. under 65)

                                                 . . .
                                                 (e.g. over 65)

18. Total number of mental health day
    hospital places   . . .

19. Average length of attendance (days)   . . .

20. What are the principal activities undertaken by nurses working in mental health day hospitals (please specify):

....

....

....

21. *Grades of staff working in mental health day hospitals* (at 31 March 1994)

	Funded establishment	In post
Grade I	. . .	. . .
Grade H	. . .	. . .
Grade G	. . .	. . .
Grade F	. . .	. . .
Grade E	. . .	. . .
Grade D1	. . .	. . .
Grade D2 (Enrolled Nurse)	. . .	. . .

Grade C   . . .   . . .
Grade B   . . .   . . .
Grade A   . . .   . . .

22. Other community facilities (at 31 March 1994; e.g.
resource centre or day centre, please specify):

....

....

....

23. Total number of places   . . .

24. Total number of appointments   . . .

25. What are the principal activities undertaken by nurses in those
     facilities:

....

....

....

26. *Grades of staff working in those facilities* (at 31 March 1994)

	Funded establishment	In post
Grade I	. . .	. . .
Grade H	. . .	. . .
Grade G	. . .	. . .
Grade F	. . .	. . .
Grade E	. . .	. . .
Grade D1	. . .	. . .
Grade D2 (Enrolled Nurse)	. . .	. . .
Grade C	. . .	. . .
Grade B	. . .	. . .
Grade A	. . .	. . .

27. *Total number of mental health secure beds* (at 31 March 1994)

Low   . . .
Medium   . . .
High   . . .

28. *Grades of staff working in secure settings* (at 31 March 1994)

	Funded establishment	In post
Grade I	. . .	. . .
Grade H	. . .	. . .
Grade G	. . .	. . .
Grade F	. . .	. . .
Grade E	. . .	. . .
Grade D1	. . .	. . .
Grade D2 (Enrolled Nurse)	. . .	. . .
Grade C	. . .	. . .
Grade B	. . .	. . .
Grade A	. . .	. . .

29. *Additional facilities* (please specify any not mentioned above)

....

....

....

Thank you for taking the time to complete the questionnaire.

Appendix 13
Postal survey of ward profiles and operational routines for acute psychiatric admission wards

To be completed by the Ward Manager or Senior Nurse in Charge

Name of NHS Trust: ....

Hospital (or other type of facility): ....

Name and telephone number (to be contact only in case of query):

....

Date : ....

Information on nursing staff

1. Please give the funded establishment (FE) and staff actually in post (IP) for the various grades of ward staff in the different catgories at 31 March 1994.

Grade	Permanent day		Permanent night		Rotate		Part-time	
	MALE FE IP	FEMALE FE IP	MALE FE IP	FEMALE FE IP	MALE FE IP	FEMALE FE IP	MALE FE IP	FEMALE FE IP
H								
G								
F								
E								
D1								
D2*								
C								
B								
A								

*Enrolled Nurse

2. Are you below the ward establishment level because of study leave, maternity leave, sickness or any other reason over the past 3 months?

    Yes

    No

3. If so, how many ward staff does this involve? ....

4. How is this issue usually resolved? By the use of:

                                                        Yes   No

    Bank nurses
    Agency nurses
    Overtime for existing staff
    Use of staff from another ward
    Other (please specify):

    ....

    ....

    ....

5. What is the rate of staff turnover per grade for the year to 31
    March 1994? (i.e. How many members of staff have left and how
    many staff have been employed in the previous 12 months?)

Grade	Turnover for year to 31 March
H	. . .
G	. . .
F	. . .
E	. . .
D1	. . .
D2 (Enrolled Nurse)	. . .
C	. . .
B	. . .
A	. . .

6. What is the usual grade mix on shifts?

	H	G	F	E	D1	D2*	B	A
Usual number on early shift								
What is the *minimum* number that can be on an early shift for safety reasons								
Usual number on late shift								
What is the *minimum* number that can be on a late shift for safety reasons								
Usual number on night shift								
What is the *minimum* number that can be on a night shift for safety reasons								
Usual number on other shifts (please specify)								

*Enrolled Nurse

7. How long has this grade mix been in operation? ....

8. What was the reason(s) for it being established? ....

    ....

9.   What is the usual gender mix on shifts?

     Early...

     Late..

     Night...

10. What is the ethnic mix on shifts (if applicable)?

     Early...

     Late..

     Night...

11. Other nurses on duty during the day (please tick one):

     Bank nurses: Always

                           Sometimes

                           Never

     Pool nurses: Always

                           Sometimes

                           Never

     Agency nurses: Always

                           Sometimes

                           Never

12. Other nurses on duty during the night (please tick one):

     Bank nurses: Always

                           Sometimes

                           Never

Pool nurses: Always

Sometimes

Never

Agency nurses: Always

Sometimes

Never

Ward meetings

13.   Do you have a regular ward community meeting between staff and patients?

Yes

No

14.   If yes, how often do these meetings take place? ....

15.   Do you have regular ward rounds involving medical staff and other professionals?

Yes

No

16.   If yes, how many per week?   . . . .

Are patients invited to attend?   . . . .

Always

Sometimes

Never

17.   Do you have other interdisciplinary meetings on this ward?

Yes

No

18.   If yes, how often (please tick one box)?

        Weekly

        Monthly

        Infrequently

19.   What is the purpose of these meetings? ....

....

Ward routines and practices

20.   Type of ward (please tick one):

        Mixed – male and female

        Male

        Female

21.   What are the shift times?

        Early day shift   ....

        Late day shift   ....

        Night shift   ....

        Other shifts (for example, twilight – please specify):

        ....

22.   Is a particular model of care practised?

        Yes

        No

23.   If yes, what is it (please specify)? ....

....

24.   Are quality measures used on the ward?

       Yes

       No

25.   If yes, what kinds (for example, audit, peer audit, etc.)?

       ....

       ....

26.   Are individual patient care plans used on the ward?

       Yes

       No

27.   If yes, how are they used (please specify)?

       ....

       ....

       ....

28.   How often are they reviewed? ....

29.   Do you have written ward nursing standards (please tick one)?

       Yes

       In preparation

       No

30.   If yes, what do they cover?

       ....

       ....

       ....

31.   Has clinical supervision of nurses by senior colleagues been introduce on this ward?

Yes

No

32.   If yes, are formal meetings held with the supervisor?

Yes

No

33.   How frequently do formal meetings take place (please tick one)?

Once a week

Once a fortnight

Once a month

Less frequently
than monthly

34.   Is all clinical supervision provided by nurses?

Yes

No

35.   If not, what other professionals provide this supervision (please tick all categories that apply)?

Occupational therapists

Psychologists

Psychiatrists

Others (please specify):...

....

36. Does your ward staff establishment include a 'link' nurse who works in the community (for example, a community mental health nurse: (CPN)?

    Yes

    No

37. Has the care programme approach (CPA) for discharge been introduced on your ward?

    Yes

    No

38. If so, when was this introduced (please give date)? ....

39. What proportion of your patients are offered CPA? ....

40. What proportion of those patients offered CPA accept the offer?......

41. Who co-ordinates the care patients receive in hospital? ....

42. Who co-ordinates the care of individuals in the community? ....

Information on patients

43. Ward bed complement   ....

44. Usual bed occupancy   ....

45. Average length of stay (weeks)   ....

46. Average number of patients on a section per week:

    Section 2   . . . .

    Section 3   . . . .

    Section 4   . . . .

    Section 5(2)   . . . .

Section 5(4)   . . . .

Section 37   . . . .

47.   Any other section (please specify):

....

....

48.   Average number of patients on a section per year:

Section 2   . . . .

Section 3   . . . .

Section 4   . . . .

Section 5(2)   . . . .

Section 5(4)   . . . .

Section 37   . . . .

49.   Any other section (please specify):

....

....

50.   Average number of patients per week suffering from:

    1.   schizophrenia   . . .

    2.   affective (mood) psychosis   . . .

    3.   depressive disorders   . . .

    4.   anxiety states   . . .

    5.   dementia   . . .

    6.   eating disorders   . . .

7.   personality disorders   . . .

8.   drug problem   . . .

9.   alcohol/substance abuse   . . .

10. child abuse or adult
     survivors of child abuse   . . .

11. social problems   . . .

12. other (please specify): ....

     ....

     ....

51. Average number of patients per week on different observation
     levels: ....

     observation 1 (nurse within touching distance of the patient at
     all times) ....

     observation 2 (nurse must be able to see the patient at all times)
     ....

     observation 3 (nurse should be informed by the patient of
     whereabouts and be on the ward at specified times)....................

     observation 4 (nurse should know the whereabouts of the
     patient) ....

52. How many patients in the following age groups are on your
     ward at present?

     Under 30   . . .

     30–50   . . .

     51–65   . . .

     Over 65   . . .

53. What is the average number of patients per week from different ethnic origins?

Asian – Bangladeshi   . . .

Asian – Chinese   . . .

Asian – Indian   . . .

Asian – Pakistani   . . .

Asian – Other   . . .   please state ....

Black – African   . . .

Black – Caribbean   . . .

Black – Other   . . .   please state ....

White   . . .

Any other ethnic group (please state):

....

54. Average number of patients who have been on an acute psychiatric admission ward before their present period in hospital?

. . . .

55. On average, what is the number of patients who are readmitted within 2 weeks of discharge?

. . . .

56. Do your patients see officials/professionals *on the ward* who are not members of the ward staff (please tick all categories that apply)?

Solicitors/legal representatives   . . . .

Social workers   . . . .

Community mental health
nurses (CPNs)   . . . .

Psychologists   . . . .

Psychotherapists   . . . .

Occupational therapists   . . . .

Advocacy   . . . .

Other health workers (please specify):.....................................

Therapy sessions

57.   Number of ECT sessions available per week (please tick one):

       One

       Two

       Three or more

       None available

58.   Average number of patients from this ward receiving ECT treat-
       ment each week:

       ....

59.   What therapies are provided by nursing staff on the ward (please
       specify the therapies provided)?

       ....

       ....

       ....

60.   What therapies are provided by other professionals on the ward
       (please specify the therapies provided)?

       ....

       ....

       ....

61. Usual number of occupational therapy sessions available per week:

     Mornings   . . . .

     Afternoons   . . . .

62. Average number of patients from this ward to go to occupational therapy each week:

     Mornings   . . . .

     Afternoons   . . . .

63. Are other therapies provided off the ward?

     Yes

     No

64. If yes, please list the type of therapy, and the usual number of patients from this ward who attend each week:

Therapy	*Patients per week*
....	....
....	....
....	....

Thank you for taking the time to complete the questionnaire.

Appendix 14 Summary reports from feedback seminars

Introduction

The issues outlined below were identified by participants who attended a feedback seminar held in Leeds on 27 February 1996. The aim of the seminar was to present the principal findings from the Department of Health-funded study: 'The Nursing Care Provided for Acute Psychiatric Patients' to representatives from participating field-work sites. What follows is a summary of site representatives' reactions to the draft findings. The study was undertaken by the Community Care Division, Nuffield Institute for Health at the University of Leeds.

Ward Management

The ward management role of G grade nurses

- If it was accepted that the most senior ward nurse had increasingly become a manager/administrator, did the ward manager need to be a nurse? Some participants suggested that the post needed to be a nurse for clinical supervision and teaching purposes.
- What were the training implications of the shift from a primarily clinical role to one that was more managerial in orientation?
- What were the support needs of the ward manager role, for example secretarial and use of IT?
- There was a view expressed that the line management and clinical supervision roles could not be undertaken by the same individual. At a number of sites, the G grade nurse undertook line management responsibilities, and F grade nurses carried out clinical supervision of staff.

Paperwork and administration

- The issue of completing paperwork was identified as a particular problem for senior staff and one which contributed to the pressures on them. However, it was not the volume of paperwork *per se* that they were required to complete but the level of *repetition* of much of it. Similar information, but in slightly different forms, was required by a number of managers. With respect to admissions, for example, information might be required by medical audit personnel, CPA managers, IT managers and purchasers.
- Much of the administration undertaken was considered *routine*; could this be more appropriately completed by others, for example A grade nursing assistants and/or secretaries?

Relationship with medical staff

- Accountability for patient care and treatment was increasingly seen as a 'shared' responsibility between medical staff and senior nursing staff. This was identified as a positive development by most participants.

Providing care

The changing focus of nursing

Caring or counselling role?

- The reported emphasis placed on acquiring counselling skills did not appear consistent with the increasingly demanding patient mix encountered on wards. Such a patient mix was seen to militate against a counselling approach. There was a need to match training needs more appropriately to the demands of patients.

Custodial or therapeutic role?

- Closely allied to the caring/counselling issue discussed above was the question of whether nursing was having to adopt a more *custodial* approach to care – owing to the demanding nature of the patient mix – in contrast to the *therapeutic* approach emphasised in nurse training and practice. The high proportion of detained patients was, in part, cited as evidence to support the shift to a more custodial approach.
- If there had been a shift to a more custodial approach, many participants felt that there was an important role for advocacy services to play as protectors of patients rights.

Spectrum of care

- Other participants felt that while the development of advocacy services was important, of much greater importance was the development of a spectrum of local services that addressed the increasingly diverse nature of individual needs. The generic acute ward may not be an appropriate structure for dealing with so diverse a range of patient problems.
- A number of participants questioned whether the *generic* mental health nurse continued to be viable and whether nursing teams should increasingly be made up of *specialist* staff appointed for their skills in dealing with particular mental health problems.
- The issue of whether the district general hospital site was always the most appropriate location for acute wards was raised.

Defensive practice

- The need to find a scapegoat if mistakes occurred meant that the public was increasingly likely to seek legal redress. This reinforced the need for *written* records and hence the volume of paperwork that was required to be completed by ward staff.

Resources

- Is there a need to examine how resources are distributed between hospital and community services?
- There is a need to examine how resources and skills are used because of the high level of staff turnover. A number of reasons were given to explain this, including discontent, more attractive opportunities, stress, staffing levels and training, and the pace of change.
- There is a need to examine issues concerned with staff recruitment and retention.

Nurse training

- Current nursing practice – with its emphasis on care planning and care management – is not adequately reflected in nurse training.
- The theory-oriented Project 2000 curriculum meant that newly qualified nurses often required additional training and supervision owing to their lack of practical skills.

Patient mix

- The greater diversity in the patient mix encountered on wards had resulted in more patient management problems for staff. It was noted that of particular concern was the rise in the admission of young men with drug and/or alcohol and psychotic problems. This had led to an increase in violent incidents on wards. A suggestion was made that there was perhaps a need to review the skill mix of staff so that it more closely reflected the needs of patients.
- The more demanding nature of the patient mix also raised the issue of whether hospitals had adequate staff counselling systems in place and whether they were transparent to staff.

The role of named nurse

- The Patients' Charter had emphasised that the nurse–patient contact should focus in particular on the care plan. One result of this emphasis had been to squeeze the time for general socialising between staff and patients, owing to pressures of work on nurses. The resultant reduction in nurse–patient contact was raised as an issue of concern by many patients.

Team working

- A *team* approach to nursing was adopted at many sites. What were the implications of such an approach for nurse accountability, skill mix and roles, stress management and training?

Paperwork and administration

- With respect to organising meetings, many participants questioned whether this was a good use of nurses' time and whether unqualified staff could take on such tasks.
- The increase in the number of sectioned patients on the ward had resulted in a greater number of appeals against such sections. The consequence of this had been an increase in paperwork for staff, as they were required to prepare reports for Mental Health Act Tribunals and/or senior managers' hearings.
- Could this be reduced by the use of IT and the development of effective audit mechanisms?

Care programme approach (CPA)

- This initiative was said to have improved communication between hospital and community staff. However, was the CPA working

effectively in all areas, or was it exacerbating the problem of bed-blocking and increasing the pressure on beds?
- The issue of the paper-intensive nature of the CPA was also raised.

Outcomes of nursing interventions

- There was a recognition among participants that it was often diffi-cult to measure the contribution made of *any* profession – in isola-tion from others – to patient recovery.
- The move to greater multidisciplinary working has raised the issue of whether nurses – or any other professionals – could be held *solely* accountable for patients if mistakes occurred.
- Health of the Nation outcome scales were identified as being of limited use because they largely ignored the social and environ-mental aspects affecting patient recovery.
- The use of clinical pathways that assign specific tasks to each profession may be a way forward. It was also suggested that their use might lead to a reduction in the amount of paperwork that must be completed by nurses.
- Questions were raised about whether the nursing process had significantly improved the quality of patient care.

Relationship with medical staff

- There was a perception that medical staff might have contributed to increased pressures on ward staff with their 'get people into hospital' approach. A number of questions were raised about this: were decisions to admit always concerned with the treatment of patients or the containment of a particular problem? Did nurses appreciate the consequences of their admis-sion decisions? Should nurses exercise a greater influence over such decisions?
- Nurses are more willing to challenge medical decisions. This was partly related to a perceived vacuum left by the poor support provided to junior medical staff.

Research and development

- Could a model – based on the present research – be developed for individual sites to use as part of service development?

SUMMARY OF ISSUES RAISED AT THE SEMINAR ON 5 JUNE 1996

Introduction

The issues outlined below were identified by participants who attended the feedback seminar held in London on 5 June 1996. The aim of the seminar was to present the principal findings from the Department of Health-funded study 'The Nursing Care Provided for Acute Psychiatric Patients' to representatives from participating fieldwork sites. The study was undertaken by the Community Care Division, Nuffield Institute for Health at the University of Leeds.

Key issues

Clarify the role of ward staff

1. G and F grade nurses

   - There was a danger that the G grade nurses might be losing their clinical role by default, in favour of their managerial/administrative responsibilities. If this is the case, it raises the issue of whether the ward manager needs to be a nurse.
   - G and F grade nurses *should* be clinical experts 'leading from the front.' Questions were raised about whether general managers and senior nurse managers are asking similar or conflicting things of G grades. There is a need to look at the systems at senior management level and how they impact on the work of senior ward staff.
   - If senior ward nurses have little clinical time, who are the role models for E and D grade nurses?
2. E and D grade nurses

   - Many nurses are seeking qualifications in counselling, but is that skill/role compatible with the pattern of care on acute wards? Is it increasingly dominated by crisis intervention?
3. A grade nursing assistants

   - The overall lack of A grade staff was noted. There was some questioning of whether unqualified staff should be involved in acute wards, except for household activities.

Staff supervision and sickness

   - The need for effective supervision was considered vital as pressure on staff increased. However, much supervision appeared *ad hoc* and unplanned. Other professions, for example social workers, occupational therapists and psychologists, insist that they receive adequate supervision. Nurses do not appear to be as reticent on this point.

- Supervision should be planned into the duty rota. Otherwise, there is a danger that it will always take second place to more urgent ward demands.
- The researchers noted that a proportion of staff confessed at interview to taking occasional days sick leave in response to pressures. Moreover, many permanent staff said that they often came in to cover for sick colleagues on their days off. Perhaps the majority of staff are doing extra hours? Senior managers *must* take the sickness and extra hours issues seriously.

Administration and paperwork

- There was increasing evidence of defensive administration: the need to cover one's back owing to a small number of severe untoward incidents.
- One site had carried out a study among their patients which found that they had only passing relationships with nurses, who were either in the office writing or dealing with incidents.
- If nurses are spending a lot of time liaising on the telephone, why not do this with patients next to them? This could prove to be an important therapeutic aspect of care planning.
- 150% bed occupancy levels means that nurses have to carry the paperwork for a larger number of people: this involves extra liaison and communication caused by many patients being on leave, sometimes taking very extended periods of leave.

Expectations

1. Nurses

  - Nurses are trained to work on a model that people enter hospital, get better and leave. Nurses may not have adapted sufficiently to the *new* way of working: that people leave hospital after their condition has been stabilised.
  - Is there a need for greater honesty with nurses, in that they may never see the end of the illness because patients move back into the community before they are fully better?

2. Patients

  - There is a need for greater honesty with patients about what they can expect when they enter hospital. They are *not* going to receive counselling from nurses, but they are going to have their symptoms controlled.

Risk assessment and management

- An element of underlying risk is always present on acute wards. The question was raised about what is an acceptable risk and whether the concept of risk had been 'stretched' because of the pressure on beds.
- Much risk management is *reactive* to incidents on the ward. The quality of *proactive* risk assessment is important in terms of what systems are in place to make informed decisions. In this context, it is important for staff to operate on the basis of evidence-based practice as this could help them to make informed risk assessments.
- There may be a need to define what proactive practice is and then pilot it on the ward to see whether or not it is possible to break the vicious circle of being only reactive rather than proactive.

Discharge and readmissions

- There are still people who are not discharged because they are waiting for suitable accommodation and who might be classified as bed-blockers. At times, this accounted for at least 25% of current inpatients.
- Concern was not merely about the 'revolving door' 6 months hence but about people who are readmitted within a few weeks, because they do not take their medication. This undermines nurses' morale.
- There was concern about the absence of a systematic approach for assessing who should be discharged: pressure on beds meant that assessments were made on the basis that someone had not created a problem for a few days rather than in terms of what support systems they had in the community.

Relationship with other health professionals

- Shared accountability was considered a mixed blessing. Too often, nurses spend much of their time chasing others about what they intend to do, particularly medical staff. This means that nurses do not have sufficient time for one-to-one work with patients, to run groups or to provide a better therapeutic environment for patients.
- The emphasis placed on teamworking, appears to be lacking outside the weekly multidisciplinary team meeting.

- There needs to be an analysis of who does what with respect to patient care, if teamworking is to prove meaningful.
- There is a need to review what medical staff, occupational therapists, psychologists and other health professionals do with patients, and to understand the inputs and outcomes that derive from others' interventions. Reviews of the nursing role are more common than those of other professionals.

Training and skills

- There had been a shift in the type of skill needed in acute wards, which raises the question of whether a different breed of nurse is needed: nurses are doing more crisis intervention.
- It is important to relate training and the skills that nurses are equipped with to the current role of an acute ward and its patient mix. The skills that are necessary, given that patients are in acute wards for relatively short periods of time, include crisis management, anger management, how to manage voices and relapse management. Nurses should be promoted on the basis of relevant skills and experience.
- More IT skills and extra clerical support may be only part of the answer to dealing with pressures. If nurses are faced with high bed occupancy levels, a higher proportion of severely ill people on wards and higher patient expectations, it raises questions about how they are trained to cope with such pressures.
- Concerns were expressed about the level of skills that newly qualified nurses bring with them on to the ward. They were not seen as appropriate to what is needed. One site had started a preceptorship model to address this problem.
- It was also questioned whether 3 years training was enough, whether nurses had sufficient contact with patients during training and whether the range and length of experiences to which they were exposed were adequate.

The suitability of generic wards as caring environments

There should be *specialist* wards that concentrate on what people's needs are rather than locality-based, generic wards. They might be split, for example, by admission, length of stay, age, sex or ethnic group.

Appendix 15
Additional data for text figures

For key to abbreviations, see relevant figure in the text.

Figure 5.1 Activities undertaken by G grade nurses during recorded observations, 1985–96 (%)

		1985–89 (%)	1990–93 (%)	1994–96 (%)
D	One-to-one	9.3	6.9	3.4
	Medication	3.6	2.3	1.6
	Observations	6.1	3.5	0.7
	Personal care	2.6	0.9	0.0
	Escort	0.3	0.2	0.0
	Recreation	7.1	3.4	0.0
	ECT	0.0	0.1	0.0
	Total	29.0	17.3	5.7
I	Ward round	14.7	11.3	6.8
	Hand-overs	16.3	14.6	9.9
	Total	31.0	25.9	16.7
A	Meetings	4.7	8.8	17.0
	Office	25.5	34.9	48.4
	Teaching	0.7	2.2	5.9
	Domestic	1.6	1.5	1.0
	Errands	0.8	0.3	0.0
	Total	33.3	47.7	72.3
P	Breaks	5.2	8.1	5.1
		98.5	99.0	99.8

Figure 5.2 Activities undertaken by F grade nurses during recorded observations, 1985–96 (%)

		1985–89 (%)	1990–93 (%)	1994–96 (%)
D	One-to-one	17.1	10.6	7.6
	Medication	4.6	4.1	7.8
	Observations	0.0	9.9	4.6
	Personal care	7.6	2.0	2.6
	Escort	0.4	0.5	0.0
	Recreation	15.0	7.0	0.0
	ECT	0.2	0.3	0.0
	Total	44.9	34.4	22.6
I	Ward round	5.6	8.2	3.9
	Hand-overs	20.1	17.7	13.3
	Relatives	0.0	0.0	9.1
	Total	25.7	25.9	26.3
A	Meetings	3.6	3.9	0.0
	Office	13.7	21.2	25.9
	Teaching	0.0	0.9	0.0
	Domestic	1.5	1.7	0.0
	Off-ward	0.0	0.0	11.6
	Errands	3.2	0.7	0.0
	Total	22.0	28.4	37.5
P	Breaks	7.6	10.5	11.9
		100.2	99.2	98.3

Figure 5.3 Activities undertaken by G grade nurses during recorded observations by region, 1994–96 (%)

		A (%)	B (%)	C (%)
D	One-to-one	1.7	3.4	7.5
	Medication	1.4	3.4	0.0
	Observations	1.7	6.7	0.0
	Total	4.8	13.5	7.5
I	Ward round	6.6	0.0	13.9
	Hand-overs	10.8	13.7	4.8

(contd)

Figure 5.3 (contd)

		A (%)	B (%)	C (%)
	Total	17.4	13.7	18.7
A	Meetings	13.3	22.3	27.7
	Office	48.7	36.3	43.3
	Teaching	8.3	5.7	2.8
	Domestic	0.0	3.4	0.0
	Total	70.3	67.7	73.8
P	Breaks	8.1	6.7	0.0
		100.6	101.6	100.0

Figure 5.4 Activities undertaken by F grade nurses during recorded observations by region, 1994–96 (%)

		A (%)	B (%)	C (%)
D	One-to-one	0.0	22.6	7.7
	Medication	9.4	12.9	3.7
	Observations	0.0	0.0	11.4
	Personal care	0.0	0.0	6.5
	Total	9.4	35.5	29.3
I	Ward round	0.0	0.0	9.8
	Hand-overs	14.0	29.0	4.9
	Relatives	22.8	0.0	0.0
	Total	36.8	29.0	14.7
A	Office	43.0	22.6	11.0
	Off-ward	0.0	0.0	29.0
	Total	43.0	22.6	44.0
P	Breaks	11.1	12.9	12.3
		100.3	100.0	100.3

Figure 5.5 Activities undertaken by G grade nurses during recorded observations by geographical location of hospital, 1994–96 (%)

		IC (%)	OU (%)	R (%)
D	One-to-one	5.7	5.2	0.0
	Group sessions	0.0	3.4	0.0
	Medication	0.0	5.2	1.5
	Observations	0.0	3.4	5.0
	Total	5.7	17.2	6.5
I	Ward round	10.4	0.0	6.6
	Hand-over	5.9	10.1	13.7
	Total	16.3	10.1	20.3
A	Meetings	4.6	6.8	22.1
	Office	43.9	43.7	42.7
	Teaching	8.9	8.6	1.5
	Domestic	0.0	5.2	0.0
	Off-ward	20.8	0.0	0.0
	Total	78.2	64.3	66.3
P	Breaks	0.0	8.9	7.0
		100.2	100.5	100.1

Figure 5.6 Activities undertaken by F grade nurses during recorded observations by geographical location of hospital, 1994–96 (%)

		IC (%)	OU (%)	R (%)
D	One-to-one	7.7	22.6	0.0
	Medication	3.7	12.9	9.4
	Personal care	6.5	0.0	0.0
	Observations	11.4	0.0	0.0
	Total	29.3	35.5	9.4
I	Ward round	9.8	0.0	0.0
	Hand-over	4.9	29.0	14.0
	Relatives	0.0	0.0	22.8
	Total	14.7	29.0	36.8
A	Office	15.0	22.6	43.0
	Off-ward	29.0	0.0	0.0

(contd)

Figure 5.6 (contd)

		IC (%)	OU (%)	R (%)
	Total	44.0	22.6	43.0
P	Breaks	12.3	12.9	11.1
		100.3	100.0	100.3

Figure 5.7 Activities undertaken by G grade nurses during recorded observations by hospital type, 1994–96 (%)

		DGH (%)	WT (%)	O (%)
D	One-to-one	4.8	0.0	3.7
	Group sessions	0.0	0.0	1.7
	Medication	2.0	0.0	2.6
	Observations	6.7	6.0	1.7
	Total	13.5	6.0	9.7
I	Ward round	8.8	0.0	10.4
	Hand-over	14.4	8.7	7.3
	Total	23.2	8.7	17.7
A	Meetings	20.0	9.4	8.0
	Office	27.0	59.3	43.6
	Teaching	2.0	0.0	13.2
	Domestic	0.0	0.0	2.6
	Off-ward	11.9	15.8	0.0
	Total	60.9	84.5	67.4
P	Breaks	2.5	6.8	5.7
		100.1	100.0	100.5

Figure 5.8 Activities undertaken by F grade nurses during recorded observations by hospital type, 1994–96

		DGH (%)	WT* (%)	O (%)
D	One-to-one	3.7	–	10.2
	Medication	3.7	–	10.5
	Observations	7.4	–	2.7
	Personal care	2.5	–	2.7
	Total	17.3		26.1
I	Ward round	9.8	–	3.0
	Hand-overs	4.9	–	19.0
	Relatives	22.8	–	0.0
	Total	37.5		22.0
A	Office	34.2	–	20.7
	Off-ward	0.0	–	19.3
	Total	34.2		40.0
P	Breaks	11.4	–	12.2
		100.4	–	100.3

*Not on duty during observations of shifts.

Figure 5.9 Activities undertaken by G grade nurses during recorded observations by bed occupancy level, 1994–96 (%)

		≥ 100 (%)	< 100 (%)	(%)
D	One-to-one	6.6	0.0	
	Medication	2.1	1.2	
	Observations	0.0	5.3	
	Total	8.7	6.5	
I	Ward round	8.3	5.3	
	Hand-overs	6.1	13.7	
	Total	14.4	19.0	
A	Meetings	21.6	18.9	
	Office	41.2	45.5	
	Teaching	10.7	1.2	
	Domestic	2.1	0.0	

(contd)

Figure 5.9 (contd)

		≥ 100	< 100
	Total	75.6	65.6
P	Breaks	2.5	7.6
		101.2	98.7

Figure 5.10 Activities undertaken by F grade nurses during recorded observations by bed occupancy level, 1994–96 (%)

		≥ 100	< 100
D	One-to-one	12.6	0.0
	Medication	6.7	9.4
	Personal care	4.3	0.0
	Observations	7.5	0.0
	Total	31.1	9.4
I	Ward round	6.5	0.0
	Hand-overs	12.9	14.0
	Relatives	0.0	22.8
	Total	19.4	36.8
A	Office	17.9	43.0
	Off-ward	19.3	0.0
	Total	37.2	43.0
P	Breaks	12.5	11.1
		100.2	100.3

Figure 6.1 Activities undertaken by E grade nurses during recorded observations, 1985–96 (%)

		1985–89	1990–93	1994–96
D	One-to-one	10.8	9.3	8.2
	Medication	6.2	8.5	11.0
	Observations	17.2	16.8	15.7
	Personal care	4.1	3.6	2.0
	Escort	2.4	1.7	0.7

(contd)

Figure 6.1 (contd)

		1985–89	1990–93	1994–96
	Recreation	10.5	3.9	1.5
	ECT	0.8	0.2	0.0
	Total	52.0	44.0	39.1
I	Ward round	3.7	4.3	6.2
	Handovers	15.4	12.2	10.1
	Relatives	0.0	0.0	0.3
	Total	19.1	16.5	16.6
A	Meetings	1.0	1.5	2.1
	Office	15.7	21.4	29.9
	Teaching	0.9	1.0	1.3
	Domestic	1.8	3.3	3.5
	Errands	0.9	0.5	0.3
	Total	20.3	27.7	37.1
P	Breaks	9.2	11.0	7.6
		100.6	99.2	100.4

Figure 6.2 Activities undertaken by D grade nurses during recorded observations, 1985–96 (%)

		1985–89	1990–93	1994–96
D	One-to-one	6.9	12.9	8.5
	Medication	5.5	4.5	4.7
	Observations	33.1	0.3	3.1
	Personal care	2.6	5.3	5.5
	Escort	3.0	5.1	5.3
	Recreation	5.9	11.4	3.0
	ECT	0.6	0.9	1.1
	Total	57.6	40.4	31.2
I	Ward round	3.0	2.2	1.4
	Hand-overs	9.8	18.4	10.8
	Relatives	0.0	0.0	0.7
	Total	12.8	20.6	12.9

(contd)

Figure 6.2 (contd)

		1985–89	1990–93	1994–96
A	Meetings	0.3	2.7	0.7
	Office	12.8	24.2	33.7
	Teaching	0.5	0.2	2.6
	Domestic	2.3	2.4	5.3
	Errands	0.6	2.6	0.0
	Total	16.5	32.1	42.3
P	Breaks	12.2	6.2	12.5
		99.1	99.3	98.9

Figure 6.3 Activities undertaken by E grade nurses during recorded observations by region, 1994–96 (%)

		A	B	C
D	One-to-one	8.5	10.7	9.6
	Medication	10.1	6.4	8.6
	Observations	4.3	15.4	26.0
	Personal care	1.6	2.0	2.7
	Escort	0.0	0.0	2.7
	Recreation	0.0	2.0	2.7
	Total	24.5	36.5	52.3
I	Ward round	6.0	9.7	1.6
	Hand-overs	13.0	7.2	10.0
	Relatives	0.0	0.0	1.1
	Total	19.0	16.9	12.7
A	Meetings	4.1	2.0	0.0
	Office	37.6	29.9	19.5
	Teaching	1.1	2.4	0.0
	Domestic	3.2	3.9	3.2
	Errands	0.0	0.0	1.1
	Total	46.0	38.2	23.8
P	Breaks	11.1	8.5	11.6
		100.6	100.1	100.4

Figure 6.4 Activities undertaken by D grade nurses during recorded observations by region, 1994–96 (%)

		A	B	C
D	One-to-one	12.1	11.8	10.1
	Group sessions	1.2	0.0	4.6
	Medication	2.7	4.0	8.3
	Observations	1.2	0.0	11.0
	Personal care	4.4	2.3	11.5
	Escort	0.0	10.7	0.0
	Recreation	6.1	2.9	0.0
	ECT	4.6	0.0	0.0
	Total	32.3	31.7	45.5
I	Ward round	4.6	0.0	1.2
	Hand-overs	14.3	11.1	6.9
	Relatives	0.0	1.4	0.0
	Total	18.9	12.5	8.1
A	Meetings	0.0	0.0	2.8
	Office	31.8	32.5	29.9
	Teaching	6.0	2.2	0.0
	Domestic	0.0	10.7	0.0
	Total	37.8	45.4	32.7
P	Breaks	11.3	10.6	13.5
		100.3	100.2	99.8

Figure 6.5 Activities undertaken by E grade nurses during recorded observations by geographical location of hospital, 1994–96 (%)

		IC	OU	R
D	One-to-one	9.0	7.8	6.7
	Group sessions	1.0	5.3	0.0
	Escort	1.6	0.0	0.0
	Recreation	1.6	0.0	2.0
	Medication	9.4	4.2	9.0
	Personal care	1.6	0.0	3.6
	Observations	18.9	13.9	12.5
	Total	43.1	38.2	31.8

(contd)

Figure 6.5 (contd)

		IC	OU	R
I	Ward round	5.7	6.3	6.7
	Hand-over	10.3	7.0	12.7
	Relatives	0.6	0.0	0.0
	Total	16.6	13.3	16.4
A	Meetings	2.0	1.4	2.6
	Office	23.2	27.9	39.2
	Teaching	0.0	4.8	1.2
	Domestic	2.9	7.7	2.1
	Errands	0.6	0.0	0.0
	Total	28.7	41.8	45.1
P	Breaks	11.6	7.0	7.1
		100.0	100.3	100.4

Figure 6.6 Activities undertaken by D grade nurses during recorded observations by geographical location of hospital, 1994–96 (%)

		IC	OU	R
D	One-to-one	12.3	17.1	9.4
	Group sessions	2.3	0.0	0.8
	Escort	0.0	0.0	14.2
	Recreation	1.6	0.0	5.7
	ECT	0.0	0.0	3.0
	Medication	5.6	0.0	5.1
	Personal care	10.3	0.0	0.8
	Observations	5.5	0.0	1.0
	Total	38.6	17.1	40.0
I	Ward round	0.6	0.0	3.0
	Hand-over	9.0	11.4	13.2
	Relatives	0.0	0.0	1.9
	Total	9.6	11.4	18.1
A	Meetings	1.4	0.0	0.0
	Office	32.4	28.6	31.7
	Teaching	2.4	0.0	3.6
	Domestic	0.0	31.4	3.8

(contd)

Figure 6.6 (contd)

		IC	OU	R
	Total	36.2	60.0	39.1
P	Breaks	15.5	11.4	2.3
		99.9	99.9	99.5

Figure 6.7 Activities undertaken by E grade nurses during recorded observations by hospital type, 1994–96 (%)

		DGH	WT	O
D	One-to-one	8.4	6.9	8.2
	Group sessions	0.0	0.0	3.9
	Medication	12.7	5.9	5.8
	Observations	12.6	20.7	15.1
	Personal care	1.0	5.1	0.8
	Escort	0.0	1.6	0.8
	Recreation	2.0	0.0	2.0
	Total	36.7	40.2	36.6
I	Ward round	6.1	6.9	5.6
	Hand-overs	14.7	5.7	6.6
	Relatives	0.0	0.0	0.8
	Total	20.8	12.6	13.0
A	Meetings	0.0	3.5	3.0
	Office	30.4	31.0	28.3
	Teaching	0.0	2.6	2.4
	Domestic	2.2	5.4	5.1
	Errands	0.0	0.0	0.8
	Total	32.6	42.5	39.6
P	Breaks	10.3	5.0	11.6
		100.4	100.3	100.8

Figure 6.8 Activities undertaken by D grade nurses during recorded observations by hospital type, 1994–96 (%)

		DGH	WT	O
D	One-to-one	11.0	9.8	14.9
	Group sessions	0.0	1.2	3.0
	Medication	7.6	4.9	1.8
	Observations	3.7	1.2	3.6
	Personal care	10.4	1.2	3.4
	Escort	1.9	18.5	0.0
	Recreation	3.8	2.9	2.2
	ECT	0.0	4.6	0.0
	Total	38.4	44.3	28.9
I	Ward round	0.0	4.6	0.8
	Hand-overs	9.5	12.6	11.0
	Relatives	0.0	2.8	0.0
	Total	9.5	20.0	11.8
A	Meetings	0.0	0.0	1.8
	Office	37.0	28.9	28.2
	Teaching	2.9	1.2	3.2
	Domestic	1.9	2.8	10.5
	Total	41.8	32.9	43.7
P	Breaks	10.4	3.3	14.0
		100.1	100.5	98.4

Figure 6.9 Activities undertaken by E grade nurses during recorded observations by bed occupancy level, 1994–96 (%)

		≥ 100	< 100
D	One-to-one	7.1	9.0
	Group sessions	1.0	1.8
	Medication	7.9	8.7
	Observations	19.5	10.0
	Personal care	1.6	2.4
	Escort	1.6	0.0
	Recreation	1.6	1.3
	Total	40.3	33.2

(contd)

Figure 6.9 (contd)

		≥ 100	< 100
I	Ward round	2.8	9.0
	Hand-overs	12.5	10.6
	Relatives	0.6	0.0
	Total	15.9	19.6
A	Meetings	2.5	2.1
	Office	24.1	34.6
	Teaching	2.0	0.6
	Domestic	3.3	3.6
	Errands	0.6	0.0
	Total	32.5	40.9
P	Breaks	12.0	6.3
		100.7	100.0

Figure 6.10 Activities undertaken by D grade nurses during recorded observations by bed occupancy level, 1994–96 (%)

		≥ 100	< 100
D	One-to-one	12.6	10.3
	Group sessions	2.3	0.6
	Medication	4.2	5.3
	Observations	5.5	0.8
	Personal care	7.4	3.5
	Escort	0.0	10.7
	Recreation	1.6	4.3
	ECT	0.0	2.3
	Total	33.6	37.8
I	Ward round	0.6	2.3
	Hand-overs	10.3	11.4
	Relatives	0.0	1.4
	Total	10.9	15.1
A	Meetings	1.4	0.0
	Office	30.2	33.2
	Teaching	2.4	2.7
	Domestic	7.9	2.8
	Total	41.9	38.7
P	Breaks	12.6	7.4
		99.0	99.0

Figure 6.11 Activities undertaken by A grade nurses during recorded observations, 1985–96 (%)

		1985–89	1990–93	1994–96
D	One-to-one	17.7	8.8	9.0
	Medication	1.6	0.6	1.4
	Observations	0.0	39.9	18.0
	Personal care	25.8	10.5	15.2
	Escort	3.9	3.1	4.1
	Recreation	23.5	9.3	8.4
	ECT	0.0	0.3	0.0
	Total	72.5	72.5	56.1
I	Ward round	0.0	0.2	0.0
	Hand-overs	6.2	6.5	4.6
	Total	6.2	6.7	4.6
A	Meetings	1.5	0.0	4.4
	Office	3.6	3.5	10.1
	Teaching	0.0	0.3	0.0
	Domestic	3.6	8.3	10.3
	Errands	3.6	1.7	4.9
	Total	12.3	13.8	29.7
P	Breaks	8.5	8.2	8.7
		99.5	101.2	99.1

Figure 6.12 Activities undertaken by A grade nurses during recorded observations by region, 1994–96 (%)

		A	B	C
D	One-to-one	6.4	9.3	3.8
	Group sessions	2.9	0.0	0.0
	Medication	1.7	1.4	0.0
	Observations	14.9	16.5	35.9
	Personal care	13.4	18.1	11.3
	Escort	6.8	2.6	0.0
	Recreation	7.8	9.6	11.4
	Total	53.9	57.5	62.4
I	Hand-overs	5.3	3.7	5.7

(contd)

Figure 6.12 (contd)

		A	B	C
A	Meetings	3.5	5.6	3.8
	Office	7.7	13.0	7.6
	Domestic duties	10.8	11.0	10.7
	Errands	9.0	2.0	0.0
	Total	31.0	31.6	22.1
P	Breaks	10.4	7.9	10.7
		100.6	100.7	100.9

Figure 6.13 Activities undertaken by A grade nurses during recorded observations by geographical location of hospital, 1994–96 (%)

		IC	OU	R
D	One-to-one	8.7	2.6	8.8
	Group sessions	0.0	0.0	2.9
	Escort	2.4	10.0	2.6
	Recreation	10.6	2.7	11.1
	Medication	1.9	1.4	1.0
	Personal care	12.8	20.2	16.9
	Observations	21.0	24.4	15.5
	Total	57.4	61.3	58.8
I	Hand-overs	4.9	6.3	3.6
A	Meetings	2.5	4.7	5.8
	Office	9.3	10.3	10.5
	Domestic	8.6	6.0	13.7
	Errands	10.2	2.7	2.0
	Total	30.6	23.7	32.0
P	Breaks	6.8	9.7	5.7
		99.7	101.0	100.1

Figure 6.14 Activities undertaken by A grade nurses during recorded observations by hospital type, 1994–96 (%)

		DGH	WT	O
D	One-to-one	7.1	5.9	2.7
	Group sessions	0.0	5.8	0.0
	Medication	1.4	2.0	0.9
	Observations	17.2	11.4	23.4
	Personal care	15.2	13.8	16.3
	Escort	0.0	5.1	9.0
	Recreation	12.8	8.9	4.2
	Total	53.7	52.9	56.5
I	Hand-overs	6.0	4.0	6.0
A	Meetings	5.9	3.9	3.1
	Office	11.7	14.0	8.0
	Domestic	12.0	14.1	8.2
	Errands	3.0	4.0	10.7
	Total	32.6	36.0	30.0
P	Breaks	8.0	6.0	7.6
		100.3	98.9	100.1

Figure 6.15 Activities undertaken by A grade nurses during recorded observations by bed occupancy level, 1994–96 (%)

		≥ 100	< 100
D	One-to-one	2.4	9.9
	Group sessions	0.0	1.9
	Medication	0.0	2.1
	Observations	28.7	12.6
	Personal care	15.9	14.9
	Escort	2.4	5.0
	Recreation	6.2	10.5
	Total	55.6	56.9
I	Hand-overs	6.0	4.0
A	Meetings	4.4	4.5
	Office	8.3	10.9
	Domestic	7.6	11.6
	Errands	8.9	2.9

(contd)

Figure 6.15 (contd)

		≥ 100	< 100
	Total	29.2	29.9
P	Breaks	9.1	9.4
		99.9	100.2

Figure 6.16 Activities undertaken by patients during recorded observations 1994–96 only (%)

D	One-to-one	2.3
	Group sessions	0.8
	Medication	0.2
	Recreation	0.7
	Total	4.0
I	Treatment	7.4
	Home	9.6
	Total	17.0
O	Students	0.2
	Recreation no staff	11.4
	Off-ward	6.4
	Visitors	3.0
	Total	21.0
P	Nothing	11.2
	TV	8.4
	Self-care	8.4
	Total	28.0
S	Sleeping	30.8
		100.8

Figure 6.17 Activities undertaken by patients during recorded observations by region, 1994–96 (%)

		A	B	C
D	One-to-one	2.8	2.1	1.8
	Group sessions	0.8	0.0	2.0
	Medication	0.0	0.0	0.8
	Recreation	0.0	1.1	1.1
	Total	3.6	3.2	5.7
I	Treatment	5.4	8.2	9.7
	Home	12.9	13.5	0.0
	Total	18.3	21.7	9.7
O	Students	0.0	0.5	0.0
	Recreation no staff	9.9	13.7	9.1
	Off-ward	6.8	8.8	2.7
	Visitors	2.7	3.0	3.6
	Total	19.4	26.0	15.4
P	Nothing	6.0	5.6	20.6
	TV	5.4	8.2	12.7
	Self-care	12.7	6.6	5.1
	Total	24.1	20.4	38.4
S	Sleeping	35.1	29.0	30.9
		100.5	100.3	100.1

Figure 6.18 Activities undertaken by patients during recorded observations by geographical location of hospital, 1994–96 (%)

		IC	OU	R
D	One-to-one	3.0	1.4	1.8
	Group sessions	1.2	1.5	0.0
	Medication	1.0	0.0	0.0
	Recreation	0.6	0.0	1.1
	Total	5.8	2.9	2.9
I	Treatment	9.7	3.9	9.2
	Home	1.5	28.5	8.4

(contd)

Figure 6.18 (contd)

		IC	OU	R
	Total	11.2	32.4	17.6
O	Students	0.4	0.0	0.0
	Recreation no staff	10.7	22.5	15.3
	Off-ward	8.5	4.2	5.0
	Visitors	3.2	0.0	4.3
	Total	22.8	26.7	24.6
P	Nothing	15.3	3.7	7.3
	TV	9.6	3.9	9.2
	Self-care	6.0	9.4	11.0
	Total	30.9	17.0	27.5
S	Sleeping	29.8	21.1	27.8
		100.5	100.1	100.4

Figure 6.19 Activities undertaken by patients during recorded observations by hospital type, 1994–96 (%)

		DGH	WT	O
D	One-to-one	1.6	1.4	3.6
	Group sessions	0.0	0.8	1.6
	Medication	0.0	0.8	0.0
	Recreation	0.7	1.6	0.8
	Total	2.3	4.6	6.0
I	Treatment	8.6	13.1	4.7
	Home	4.5	2.9	14.2
	Total	13.1	16.0	18.9
O	Students	0.5	0.0	0.0
	Recreation no staff	14.4	12.7	13.0
	Off-ward	5.8	2.9	4.2
	Visitors	3.0	4.0	2.3
	Total	23.7	19.6	19.5

(contd)

Figure 6.19 (contd)

		DGH	WT	O
P	Nothing	12.5	10.7	10.8
	TV	8.6	13.1	8.1
	Self care	8.6	7.8	8.7
	Total	29.7	31.6	27.6
S	Sleeping	31.9	29.5	27.8
		100.7	101.3	99.8

Figure 6.20 Activities undertaken by patients during recorded observations by bed occupancy level, 1994–96 (%)

		≥ 100	< 100
D	One-to-one	2.3	2.2
	Group sessions	1.2	0.5
	Medication	0.5	0.0
	Recreation	0.6	0.8
	Total	4.6	3.5
I	Treatment	10.1	7.0
	Home	9.3	9.8
	Total	19.4	16.8
O	Students	0.0	0.3
	Recreation no staff	7.0	20.5
	Off-ward	6.0	6.8
	Visitors	2.8	3.2
	Total	15.8	30.8
P	Nothing	15.8	4.9
	TV	10.1	7.0
	Self care	4.9	11.4
	Total	30.8	23.3
S	Sleeping	30.7	26.2
		101.3	100.6

Bibliography

Alberg C, Bingley W, Bowers L *et al.* (1996) Learning Materials on Mental Health: Risk Assessment. Manchester: University of Manchester/Department of Health.

Altschul A (1972) Patient–Nurse Interactions: A Study of Interaction Patterns in Acute Psychiatric Wards. Edinburgh: Churchill Livingstone.

Ashworth PD, Longmate MA, Morrison P (1992) Patient participation: its meaning and significance in the context of caring. Journal of Advanced Nursing 17: 1430–9.

Audit Commission (1986) Making a Reality of Community Care. London: HMSO.

Audit Commission (1991) The Virtue of Patients: Making Best Use of Ward Nursing Resources. London: Audit Commission.

Audit Commission (1994) Finding a Place: A Review of Mental Health Services for Adults. London: HMSO.

Barnes M, Bowl M, Fisher M (1990) Sectioned: Social Services and the 1983 Mental Health Act. London: Routledge.

Beardshaw V, Robinson R (1990) New for Old – Proposals for Nursing in the 1990s. Report No. 8. London: King's Fund Institute.

Beck A (1976) Cognitive Therapy and the Emotional Disorders. London: Penguin.

Benner P (1984) From Novice to Expert: Excellence and Power in Clinical Nursing Practice. California: Addison Wesley.

Bergman R (1981) Accountability: definition and dimensions. International Nursing Review 28: 53–9.

Biehal N (1993) Changing practice: participation, rights and community care. British Journal of Social Work 23: 443–58.

Blom-Cooper L, Hally H, Murphy E (1995) The Falling Shadow: One Patient's Mental Health Care 1978–1993. London: Duckworth.

Bond S, Thomas L (1991) Issues in measuring outcomes of nursing. Journal of Advanced Nursing 16(11): 1492–502.

Bond S, Fall M, Thomas L, Fowler P, Bond J (1990) Primary Nursing and Primary Medical Care: A Comparative Study in Community Hospitals. Report No. 39. Newcastle: Health Care Research Unit, University of Newcastle.

Bottomley V (1994) Reply for Mrs Bottomley. Psychiatric Bulletin 18(7): 387–8.

Briggs A (Chairman) (1972) Report of the Committee on Nursing. Cmnd 5115. London: HMSO.

Broughton M, Divall P (1994) Care programme approach: the experience in Bath. Psychiatric Bulletin 18(10): 77–9.

Buchan J (1992) Flexibility or Fragmentation?: Trends and Prospects in Nurses' Pay. Briefing Paper No. 13. London: King's Fund Institute.

Burdock MB, Stuart GW and Lewis LD (1994) Measuring nursing outcomes in a psychiatric setting. Issues in Mental Health Nursing 15(2): 137–48.

Burnard P (1985) Learning Human Skills – an Experiential Guide for Nurses. London: Butterworth.

Burnard P (1987a) Sharing a viewpoint. Senior Nurse 7(3): 38–9.

Burnard P (1987b) Meaningful dialogue. Nursing Times 83(20): 43–5.

Butler T (1993) Changing Mental Health Services: The Politics and Policy. London: Chapman & Hall.

Caldicott F (1994a) Supervision registers: the College's response. Psychiatric Bulletin 18(7): 385–6.

Caldicott F (1994b) Update following the meeting of the Executive and Finance Committee, 4 June 1994. Psychiatric Bulletin 18(7): 388.

Carpenter P (1989) A Re-appraisal of Towell's 'Understanding Psychiatric Nursing'. Eastbourne: Sussex Downs School of Nursing.

Carson D (1991) Risk taking in mental disorder. In Carson D (Ed) Risk Taking in Mental Disorder: Analyses, Policies and Practical Strategies. Chichester: SLE Publications.

Carson D (1994) Dangerous people: through a broader conception of 'risk' and 'danger' to better decisions. Expert Evidence 3: 51–69.

Chalmers H (1995) Accountability in nursing models and the nursing process. In Watson R (Ed) Accountability in Nursing Practice. London: Chapman & Hall.

Clarke J Macleod, Hopper L, Jeeson A (1991) Progression to counselling. Nursing Times 87(8): 41–3.

Clinical Standards Advisory Group (1995a) Schizophrenia: Protocol for Assessing Services for People with Severe Mental Illness, Volume 1. London: HMSO.

Clinical Standards Advisory Group (1995b) Schizophrenia: Protocol for Assessing Services for People with Severe Mental Illness, Volume 2. London: HMSO.

Clinton M (1985) Training psychiatric nurses: why theory into practice won't go. In Altschul A (Ed) Psychiatric Nursing. London: Churchill Livingstone.

Coid JW (1993) Quality of life for patients detained in hospital. British Journal of Psychiatry 162: 611–20.

Collister B (Ed) (1988) Psychiatric Nursing Person-to-Person. London: Edward Arnold.

Cormack D (1976) Psychiatric Nursing Observed. London: Whitefriars Press.

Cormack D (1983) Psychiatric Nursing Described. London: Churchill Livingstone.

Danziger SK (1978) The issues of expertise in doctor–patient encounters during pregnancy. Social Science and Medicine 12: 359–67.

Darley MA (1995) Clinical supervision: the view from the top. Nursing Management 2(1): 14–15.

Davidge M, Elias S, Jayes R, Wood K, Yates J (1993) Survey of English Mental Illness Hospitals March 1993. Birmingham: Inter-Authority Comparisons and Consultancy.

Davidge M, Elias S, Jayes R, Wood K, Yates J (1994) Survey of English Mental Illness Hospitals March 1994: Monitoring the Closure of the 'Water Towers'. Birmingham: Inter-Authority Comparisons and Consultancy.

Davis A, Horobin G (Eds) (1977) Medical Encounters: The Experience of Illness and Treatment. London: Croom Helm.

Department of Health (1989) Caring for People. London: HMSO.

Department of Health (1990a) Caring for People: Community Care in the Next Decade and Beyond – Policy Guidance. London: HMSO.

Department of Health (1990b) The CPA for People with a Mental Illness Referred to the Specialist Psychiatric Services. Circular HC(90)/LASSL(90)11. London: DoH.

Department of Health (1990c) NHS Workforce in England. London: DoH.

Department of Health (1991) Residential Accommodation for Mentally Ill People and People with Learning Disabilities. London: DoH.

Department of Health (1992a) The Health of the Nation. London: HMSO.

Department of Health (1992b) Bed Availability for England 1991–92. London: DoH.

Department of Health (1992c) The Patient's Charter. London: HMSO.

Department of Health (1993) The Health of the Nation: Key Area Handbook – Mental Illness. London: HMSO.

Department of Health (1994a) Working in Partnership: A Collaborative Approach to Care (Butterworth Report). London: HMSO.

Department of Health (1994b) The Report of the Inquiry into the Care and Treatment of Christopher Clunis (Ritchie Report). London: HMSO.

Department of Health (1994c) Risk Assessment and Management. HSG (94)29/LASSL(94)4. London: DoH.

Department of Health (1995a) Mental Health (Patients in the Community) Act. London: HMSO.

Department of Health (1995b) Building Bridges: A Guide to Arrangements for Inter-Agency Working for the Care and Protection of Severely Mentally Ill People. London: DoH.

Department of Health (1996a) Mental Health Problems: The Spectrum of Care. London: DoH.

Department of Health (1996b) Seeing the Wood, Sparing the Trees: The Efficiency Scrutiny into the Burdens of Paperwork in NHS Trusts and Health Authorities. London: HMSO.

Department of Health and Social Security (1968) Report of the Committee on Local Authority and Allied Personal Services (Seebohm Report). Cmnd 3703. London: HMSO.

Department of Health and Social Security (1969) Report of the Committee of Inquiry into Allegations of Ill-treatment at the Ely Hospital, Cardiff. Cmnd 3795. London: HMSO.

Department of Health and Social Security (1972) Report of the Committee of Inquiry into Whittingham Hospital. Cmnd 4861. London: HMSO.

Department of Health and Social Security (1973) Report of the Committee of Inquiry into South Ockendon Hospital. HC 124. London: HMSO.

Department of Health and Social Security (1975) Better Services for the Mentally Ill. Cmnd 6233. London: HMSO.

Department of Health and Social Security (1983) The Mental Health Act London: HMSO.

Department of Health/Social Services Inspectorate (1994) The Health of the Nation – Key Area Handbook: Mental Illness, 2nd edn. London: HMSO.

Dickson G (1995) Principles of risk management. Quality in Health Care 4(2): 75–9.

Duff L (1995) Standards of care, quality assurance and accountability. In Watson R (Ed) Accountability in Nursing Practice. London: Chapman & Hall.

Engledow P (1987) Psychotherapeutic skills in nursing. Senior Nurse 7(3): 40–1.

Eriksen LR (1987) Patient satisfaction: an indicator of nursing quality. Nursing Management 18(7): 31–5.

Evans A(1993) Accountability: a core concept for primary nursing. Journal of Advanced Nursing 21: 231–4.

Fairlie A (1992) Nurse–patient communication barriers. Senior Nurse 12(3): 40–3.

Faulkner A, Field V, Muijen M (1994) A Survey of Adult Mental Health Services. London: Sainsbury Centre for Mental Health.

Flannigan CB, Glover GR, Wing JK (1994) Inner London collaborative audit of admission in two health districts. Part III: Reasons for acute admission to psychiatric wards. British Journal of Psychiatry 165(6): 750–9.

Fowler J (1996) The organisation of clinical supervision within the nursing profession: a review of the literature. Journal of Advanced Nursing 23(3): 471–8.

Geoghegan J (1995) Caring and sharing. Health Service Journal 23 November: 33–4.

Gijbels H (1995) Mental health nursing skills in an acute admissions environment: perceptions of mental health nurses and other mental health professionals. Journal of Advanced Nursing 21(3): 460–75.

Gijbels H, Burnard P (1995) Exploring the Skills of Mental Health Nurses. Aldershot: Avebury.

Glenister D (1994) Patient participation in psychiatric services: a literature review and proposal for a research strategy. Journal of Advanced Nursing 19(4): 802–11.

Goddard HA, Goddard GC (1955) The Work of the Mental Nurse (Joint Committee of the Manchester Regional Hospital Board and the University of Manchester Mental Nursing Survey). Manchester: University of Manchester.

Goffman E (1961) Asylums. Harmondsworth: Penguin.

Gournay K (1994) Redirecting the emphasis to serious mental illness. Nursing Times 90(25): 40–1.

Grantham G, Biley F (1988) Primary nursing – it really works. Nursing Standard 1(3): 30–1.

Griffiths R (1983) NHS Management Inquiry. London: HMSO.

Griffiths R (1988) Community Care: Agenda for Action. London: HMSO.

Grounds A (1995) Risk assessment and management in clinical context. In Crichton J (Ed) Psychiatric Patient Violence – Risk and Response. London: Duckworth.

Hamer S (1996) Shop around for the best education . Nursing Management 7(10): 16–17.

Handy J (1991) Stress and contradiction in psychiatric nursing. Human Relations 44(1): 39–53.

Hewison A (1995) Nurses' power in interactions with patients. Journal of Advanced Nursing 21(1): 75–82.

Heymann TD, Culling W (1994) The Patient-focused Approach: A Better Way To Run a Hospital? Kingston-upon-Thames: Kingston Hospital NHS Trust.

Heymann TD, Hallam CE, Strickland ID, Jackson RRP (1994) The Kingston Case Notes System – A Multi-disciplinary Electronic Patient Record. Kingston-upon-Thames: Kingston Hospital NHS Trust.

Higgins R (1993) Evaluation of the Richmond Fellowship Advocacy Project. Wakefield Project Paper No. 2. Leeds: Nuffield Institute for Health.

Higgins R, Wistow G (Eds) (1994) Community Care: The Developing Agenda. Report No. 5. Leeds: Nuffield Institute for Health.

Higgins R, Oldman C, Hunter DJ (1994) Let's work together: collaboration between health and social services. Health and Social Care in the Community 2(1): 279–87.

Higgins R, Hurst K, Wistow G (1995a) The Mental Health Nursing Care Provided for Acute Psychiatric Patients: Report on the Yorkshire Sites. Leeds: Nuffield Institute for Health.

Higgins R, Hurst K, Wistow G (1995b) The Mental Health Nursing Care Provided for Acute Psychiatric Patients: Comparison of Findings Between the Yorkshire and Northern Sites. Leeds: Nuffield Institute for Health.

Higgins R, Hurst K, Wistow G, Henderson M (1996a) The Nursing Care Provided for Acute Psychiatric Patients: Summary Report for Region One. Leeds: Nuffield Institute for Health.

Higgins R, Hurst K, Wistow G, Henderson M (1996b) The Nursing Care Provided for Acute Psychiatric Patients: Summary Report for Region Two. Leeds: Nuffield Institute for Health.

Higgins R, Hurst K, Wistow G, Henderson M (1996c) The Nursing Care Provided for Acute Psychiatric Patients: Summary Report for Region Three. Leeds: Nuffield Institute for Health.

Higgins R, Hurst K, Wistow G, Henderson M (1996d) The Nursing Care Provided for Acute Psychiatric Patients: Summary of Issues Raised at the February 1996 Seminar. Leeds: Nuffield Institute for Health.

Higgins R, Hurst K, Wistow G, Henderson M (1996e) The Nursing Care Provided for Acute Psychiatric Patients: Summary of Issues Raised at the June 1996 Seminar. Leeds: Nuffield Institute for Health.

Hogston R (1995) Quality nursing care: a qualitative enquiry. Journal of Advanced Nursing 21(1): 116–24.

Hollander D, Slater MS (1994) 'Sorry no beds': a problem for acute psychiatric admissions. Psychiatric Bulletin 18(9): 532–4.

Hopton J (1995) Control and restraint in contemporary psychiatric nursing: some ethical considerations. Journal of Advanced Nursing 22(1): 110–15.

House of Commons Health Committee (1994) Better off in the Community? The Care of People who are Seriously Mentally Ill. Volume 1: Session 1993–94. London: HMSO.

Howard D (1992) What makes a good psychiatric nurse? Nursing Times 88(7): 47.

Hughes G (1990) Trends in guardianship usage following the Mental Health Act 1983. Health Trends 22: 145–7.

Hurst K (1993a) Nursing Workforce Planning. London: Longman.

Hurst K (1993b) Problem Solving in Nursing Practice. London: Baillière Tindall.

Hurst K (1995a) Nursing Establishment and Skill Mix in Northern Ireland: Making the Best Use of the Mental Health Nursing Resources in the Province. Leeds: Nuffield Institute for Health.

Hurst K (1995b) Progress with Patient-focused Care in the United Kingdom. Leeds: NHSE/Nuffield Institute for Health.

Hurst K (1995c) Promotions and relegations in the psychiatric nursing league. Journal of Nursing Management 3(4): 43–6.

Hurst K, Quinn H (1992) Nursing Establishment and Skill Mix in Northern Ireland: Making the Best Use of Resources. Leeds: Nuffield Institute for Health.

Hurst K, Dean A, Trickey S (1991) The recognition and non-recognition of problem-solving stages in nursing practice. Journal of Advanced Nursing 16: 1444–55.

Hydes J (1995) Sisters under stress. Nursing Management 2(7): 10–11.

Jack B (1995) Using the named nurse system to improve patient care. Nursing Times 91(44): 30–1.

Jarrett N, Payne S (1995) A selective review of the literature on nurse–patient communication: has the patient's contribution been neglected? Journal of Advanced Nursing 22(1): 72–8.

Jewell SE (1994) Patient participation: what does it mean to nurses? Journal of Advanced Nursing 19(3): 433–8.

John AL (1961) A Study of the Psychiatric Nurse. London: ES Livingstone.

Johnson S, Thornicroft G (1995) Emergency psychiatric services in England and Wales. British Medical Journal 311(7000): 287–8.

Jones A (1990) Focus on ward managers. Senior Nurse 10(9): 4–5.

Jones K (1972) A History of Mental Health Services. London: Routledge & Kegan Paul.

Kelsey A (1995) Outcome measures: Problems and opportunities for public health nursing. Journal of Nursing Management 3(4): 25–9.

Kingdom D (1994) Care programme approach: recent government policy and legislation. Psychiatric Bulletin 18(10): 68–70.

Kirby SD, Pollock L (1995) The relationship between a medium secure environment and occupational stress in forensic psychiatric nurses. Journal of Advanced Nursing 22(5): 862–7.

Kitson AL (1986) Indicators of quality in nursing care: an alternative approach. Journal of Advanced Nursing 11(2): 133–44.

King's Fund (1993) Reshaping Mental Health Services: Implications for Britain of US Experience. London: King's Fund Institute.

Knapp M, Cambridge P, Thomason C, Beecham J, Allen C, Darton R (1992) Care in the Community: Challenge and Demonstration. Aldershot: Ashgate.

Kubsch SM (1996) Conflict, enactment, empowerment: conditions of independent therapeutic nursing interventions. Journal of Advanced Nursing 23(1): 192–200.

Laing Management Consultancy (1991) Laing's Review of Private Health Care. London: Laing.

Leary J, Gallagher T, Carson J, Fagin L, Bartlett H, Brown D (1995) Stress and coping strategies in community psychiatric nurses: a Q-methodological study. Journal of Advanced Nursing 21(2): 230–7.

Lelliott P, Audini B, Knapp M, Chisholm D (1996) The mental health residential care study: classification of facilities and description of residents. British Journal of Psychiatry 169: 139–47.

Lewis FM, Batey MV (1982a) Clarifying autonomy and accountability in the nursing service. Part 1. Journal of Nursing Administration 12(9): 13–18.

Lewis FM, Batey MV (1982b) Clarifying autonomy and accountability in nursing services. Part 2. Journal of Nursing Administration 12(10): 10–15.

Lipsedge M (1995) Clinical risk management in psychiatry. Quality in Health Care 4(2): 122–8.

McDonald A, Taylor M (1995) The Mental Health Act 1983: the application of the Act: admission to hospital and emergency intervention. Elders 4(1): 27–36.

McElroy A, Carden V, McLeish K (1995) Developing care plan documentation: an action research project. Journal of Nursing Management 3(4): 193–200.

MacFarlane J, Castledine G (1982) A Guide to the Practice of Nursing Using the

Nursing Process. London: CV Mosby.

MacIlwaine H (1983) The communication patterns of female neurotic patients with nursing staff in psychiatric units of general hospitals. In Wilson-Barnett J (Ed) Nursing Research: Ten Studies of Patient Care. Chichester: John Wiley & Sons.

McIver S (1991) Obtaining the Views of Users of Mental Health Services. London: King's Fund Centre.

McKeown M (1995) The transformation of nurses' work? Journal of Nursing Management 3(2): 67–74.

McMahon R (1988) Who's afraid of nursing care plans? Nursing Times 84(29): 39–41.

McMahon R (1991) Therapeutic nursing: theory, issues and practice. In McMahon R, Pearson A (Eds) Nursing as Therapy. London: Chapman & Hall.

MacVicar R, Swan J (1992) Theory into practice. Nursing Times 88(12): 38–40.

Malone G (1995) Letter: Mental Health Services. London: Department of Health.

Mangan P (1993) Rights and responsibilities ... ward management. Nursing Times 89(12): 66.

Marriner-Tomey A (1988) Guide to Nursing Management. St Louis: CV Mosby.

Martin FW (1984) Between the Acts: Community Mental Health Services 1959–1983. London: Nuffield Provincial Hospital Trust.

Matthews B (1995) Introducing the CPA to a multidisciplinary team: the impact on clinical practice. Psychiatric Bulletin 19(3): 143–4.

Mead D (1990) An evaluation tool for primary nursing. Nursing Standard 6(1): 37–9.

Mental Health Act Commission (1995) Sixth Biennial Report, 1993–1995. London: HMSO.

Mental Health Foundation (1994) Creating Community Care: Report of the Mental Health Foundation Inquiry into Community Care for People with Severe Mental Illness. London: MHF.

Mental Health Task Force (1994) Local Systems of Support: A Framework for Purchasing for People with Severe Mental Health Problems. London: DoH.

Mills C (1995) Evaluation of primary nursing in a nursing development unit. Nursing Times 91(39): 34–7.

Ministry of Health (1954) Report of the Committees on Internal Administration of Hospitals (Bradbeer Report). London: HMSO.

Ministry of Health (1956) Report of the Committee of Enquiry into the Cost of the National Health Service. London: HMSO.

Ministry of Health (1962) The Hospital Plan. London: HMSO.

Ministry of Health (1968) Psychiatric Nursing: Today and Tomorrow. London: HMSO.

Monaghan J (1993) Mental disorder and violence: another look. In Hodgins S (Ed) Mental Disorder and Crime. London: Sage.

Moore B (1995) Risk Assessment: A Practitioner's Guide to Predicting Harmful Behaviour. London: Whiting & Birch.

Morris P (1969) Put Away. London: Routledge & Kegan Paul.

Moss F (1995) Risk management and quality of care. Quality in Health Care 4(2): 102–7.

National Health Service Executive (1994) Introduction of Supervision Registers for Mentally Ill People from 1 April 1994. HSG(94)5. London: NHSE.

National Health Service Executive (1996) 24 Hour Nursing Care for People with Severe and Enduring Mental Health Problems. Leeds: NHSE.

Naylor MD, Munro BH, Brooten DA (1991) Measuring the effectiveness of nursing practice. Clinical Nurse Specialist 5(4): 210–15.

Netten A, Beecham J (Eds) (1993) Costing Community Care: Theory and Practice. Aldershot: Ashgate.

Nolan P (1990) Psychiatric nursing – the first 100 years. Senior Nurse 10(10): 20–3.

Nolan P (1991a) Looking at the first 100 years. Senior Nurse 11(1): 22–5.

Nolan P (1991b) Psychiatric nursing: the first 100 years. Senior Nurse 11(2): 12–14.

Nolan P (1991c) Psychiatric nursing – the first 100 years. Senior Nurse 11(3): 30–2.

Nolan PW (1993) A history of the training of asylum nurses. Journal of Advanced Nursing 18: 1193–1201.

North C, Ritchie J, Ward K (1993) Factors Influencing the Implementation of the Care Programme Approach. London: HMSO.

Northcott N (1996) Supervision to grow. Nursing Management 2(10): 18–19.

Oppenheim AM, Eeman B (1955) The Function and Training of Mental Nurses. London: Chapman & Hall.

Orton P (1996) Stress in health care professionals. British Journal of Health Care Management 2(2): 91–6.

Palmer AM (1993) Management development and the changing role of the ward manager. Journal of Nursing Management 1(1) (suppl.).

Pearson A (Ed) (1987) Nursing Quality Measurement: Quality Assurance Methods for Peer Review. Chichester: John Wiley & Sons.

Peplau HE (1952) Interpersonal Relations in Nursing. New York: GP Putnam.

Pickering M, Fox P (1987) The ward manager. Health Care Management 2(3): 23–6.

Pilgrim D, Rogers A (1993) A Sociology of Mental Health and Illness. Buckingham: Open University Press.

Porter S (1993) The determinants of psychiatric nursing practice: a comparison of sociological perspectives. Journal of Advanced Nursing 18(10): 1559–66.

Potts J (1995) Risk assessment and management: a home office perspective. In Crichton J (Ed) Psychiatric Patient Violence – Risk and Response. London: Duckworth.

Powell G, Caan W, Crowe M (1994) What events precede violent incidents in psychiatric hospitals? British Journal of Psychiatry 165: 107–12.

Powell RB, Hollander D, Tobionsky RI (1995) Crisis in admission beds. A four year survey of the bed state of Greater London's acute psychiatric units. British Journal of Psychiatry 167: 765–9.

Puri B, Rose G, Bermingham D (1992) Emergency admissions under Section 4 of the Mental Health Act: reasons for a high rate. Health Trends 24: 85-88.

Raphael W (1974) Just an Ordinary Patient: A Preliminary Survey of Opinions in Psychiatric Units in General Hospitals. London: King's Fund.

Raphael W, Peters V (1972) Psychiatric Hospitals Viewed by their Patients. London: King's Fund.

Read S (1995) Catching the Tide: New Voyages in Nursing. Sheffield: Sheffield Centre for Health and Related Research, Sheffield University.

Reed J (1995) Leadership in mental health services: what role for doctors? Psychiatric Bulletin 19(2): 67–72.

Reynolds W, Cormack D (Eds) (1990) Psychiatric and Mental Health Nursing. London: Chapman & Hall.

Richards DA, Lambert P (1987) The nursing process: the effect on patients' satisfaction with nursing care. Journal of Advanced Nursing 2(4): 559–62.

Rix G (1987) Staff sickness and its relationship to violent incidents on a regional secure unit. Journal of Advanced Nursing 12(2): 66–78.

Robb B (1967) Sans Everything. London: Nelson.

Roberts IL (1994) The health care assistants: professional supporter or budget necessity? International Journal of Health Care Quality Assurance 7(6): 20–5.

Roberts J (1993) The G grade ward sister: clinical expert and ward manager. British Journal of Nursing 2(4): 242–7.

Robinson D (1995) Are nurses fulfilling their proper role? Measuring culture trends in mental health nursing care. Psychiatric Care 2(1): 27–31.

Rodgers S (1995) Accountability in primary nursing. In Watson R (Ed) Accountability in Nursing Practice. London: Chapman & Hall.

Rogers A, Pilgrim D, Lacy R (1993) Experiencing Psychiatry: Users' Views of Services. London: Macmillan.

Roper N, Logan W, Tierny A (1980) The Elements of Nursing. Edinburgh: Churchill Livingstone.

Roy C (1984) Introduction to Nursing: An Adaptation Model. London: Prentice Hall.

Royal College of Nursing (1992) Skill Mix and Reprofiling: A Guide for RCN Members. London: RCN.

Samson C (1995) The fracturing of medical dominance in British psychiatry? Sociology of Health and Illness 17(2): 245–68.

Savage J (1995) Political implications of the named nurse concept. Nursing Times 91(41): 36–7.

Schneider J (1993) A Brief Summary of PSSRU Findings Concerning the Care Programme Approach. Canterbury: PSSRU, University of Kent.

Schutz A (1964) The well informed citizen: an essay on the social distribution of knowledge. In Broderson A (Ed) Collected Papers II. The Hague: Martinus Nijhoff.

Seed A (1994) Patients to people. Journal of Advanced Nursing 19(7): 738–48.

Shields PJ, Morrison P, Hart D (1988) Consumer satisfaction on a psychiatric ward. Journal of Advanced Nursing 13(3): 396–400.

Skelton R (1994) Nursing and empowerment: concepts and strategies. Journal of Advanced Nursing 19(3): 415–23.

Smith L (1988) Far to go? Nursing Times 84(27): 30–2.

Snowdon S (1995) Empowering the E grades. Nursing Management 2(5): 16–17.

Social Services Inspectorate (1995) Social Services Departments and the CPA: An Inspection. London: SSI/Department of Health.

Southwell M, Wistow G, Harding L (1993) The Hospital In-Patient Night. Leeds: Nuffield Institute for Health.

Spicer P, Anderson I, Freeman R, McGilp R (1995) Pathways through psychiatric care: the experience of psychiatric patients. Health and Social Care in the Community 3(6): 343–52.

Stewart N (1993) Contact point … ward management has become the central issue facing ward sisters today. Nursing Times 89(12): 65.

Thomas C, Bartlett A, Mezey GC (1995) The extent and effect of violence among psychiatric in-patients. Psychiatric Bulletin 19(10): 600–4.

Thomas LH, Bond S (1990) Towards defining the organisation of nursing care. Journal of Advanced Nursing 15(9): 1106–12.

Thomas LH, McColl E, Priest J, Bond S, Boys RJ (1996) Newcastle satisfaction with nursing scales: an instrument for quality assessments of nursing care. Quality in Health Care 5(2): 67–72.

Thornicroft G, Strathdee G (1994) How many psychiatric beds? British Medical Journal 309(6960): 970–1.

Tooth GC, Brooke (1961) Trends in the mental hospital population and their effect on future planning. Lancet 1: 710–13.

Towell D (1975) Understanding Psychiatric Nursing. London: RCN.

Trnobranski PH (1994) Nurse–patient negotiation: assumption or reality? Journal of Advanced Nursing 19(7): 733–7.

United Kingdom Central Council for Nursing, Midwifery and Health Visiting (1986) Project 2000: A New Preparation for Practice. London: UKCC.

United Kingdom Central Council for Nursing, Midwifery and Health Visiting (1987) Project 2000: The Final Proposals. London: UKCC.

United Kingdom Central Council for Nursing, Midwifery and Health Visiting (1996) Position Statement on Clinical Supervision for Nursing and Health Visiting. London: UKCC.

Vincent C, Moss F (1995) Clinical risk management, one piece of the quality jigsaw. Quality in Health Care 4(2): 73–4.

Vinestock M (1996) Risk assessment. 'A word to the wise?' Advances in Psychiatric Treatment 2: 3–10.

Wainwright P, Brimelow A, Campen Y (1986) Ward management: more than just managing. Nursing Times 82(46): 30–2.

Ward K (1988) Not just the patient in bed 3. Nursing Times 84(28): 39–40.

Watson R (Ed) (1995) Accountability in Nursing Practice. London: Chapman & Hall.

Webster L, Dean C, Kessel N (1987) Effect of the 1983 Mental Health Act on the management of psychiatric patients. British Medical Journal 295(12): 1529–32.

Woodley Team Report (1995) Report of the Independent Review Panel to East London and The City Health Authority and Newham Council, Following a Homicide in July 1994 by a Person Suffering with a Severe Mental Illness. London: East London and The City Health Authority/Newham Council.

Workman BA (1996) An investigation into how the health care assistants perceive their role as 'support workers' to qualified staff. Journal of Advanced Nursing 23(3): 612–19.

Wright S (1995) The named nurse initiative: what is the point? Nursing Times 91(47): 32–3.

Index

administration and paperwork 28,
    88–92, 150, 156, 275, 277, 280
  and CPAs 143–4
  and defensive practice 276, 280
  with difficult patient populations 64
  effect on nurse-patient contact 63–4,
    84, 113–22
admission 23–4, 94–5
  nursing assistants role 126
  pre-admission assessments 151
  pre-admission unit 96
  procedures 98–9
  re-admission 53, 281
  role of nurses 87, 96–7, 98, 99
aftercare *see* discharge and aftercare
age of patients 52–3, 60, 61
alcohol abuse 53–4, 95, 157
anger management 149, 150, 157, 282
assessment
  on admission 24, 105
  for discharge/CPA 141, 142, 281
  pre-admission assessment 151
  see also risk assessment
associate nurse 73
associated work activities 38, 79–80,
    113–27, 152
  see also administration and paperwork

Beck's Depressive Inventory Scale 105
bed occupancy levels
  1990 17
  average in fieldwork sites 33
  and direct patient care 82–3, 118–20
  and paperwork 89

and patient activities 136, 138
and patient populations 47–53, 147
RCP recommended average 17
and severely ill patients 55
strategies for over-full wards 47–8
bed provision
  division into long-stay and short-stay
    15
  national decline 16–18, 159–62
  national figures 30–1
  numbers in fieldwork sites 1988/89
    and 1991/92 30–1, 32
  relative to regional population 160
  rising demand in the 1980s 17
  see also local authorities, private sector
benefits of in-patient stays 97–8
Better off in the Community? (1994) 17

care
  checks on quality 133
  custodial or therapeutic? 64, 275
  four main aspects 24–5, 105
  nursing contribution to 132–3
  patients' perceptions of 133–5, 154
care plans 24, 106–7
  and counselling role of nurse 110
  and difficult patient populations 63,
    64
  evaluation 25, 107
  patients' understanding of 134
  role of nursing assistant 126, 127
  updating 113–22
Care Programme Approach *see* CPA
clinical supervision 77, 149–50, 156

community care, shift towards 14–18
community psychiatric nurses (CPNs)
    31, 162–3, 167
community services
    interaction with hospital services 112,
        153, 156, 276
    role in admissions 95
confidentiality 34, 235
cost of community v. hospital care 15,
    16
cost of training 131
counselling role of nurses *see under* nurse
    roles
counselling for staff 77–8, 277
CPA (Care Programme Approach)
    141–5, 277–8
    national introduction 16, 27–8
    nurses' role 142, 143, 144, 145, 151,
        152, 153
    patients' perceptions of 144–5
    suggested tiered 144
crisis management 63, 75, 149, 150, 282

D/E grade nurses 108, 113–22, 151–2,
    279
    see also named nurse
defensive practice 152, 156–7, 157, 276,
    280
detained patients 26, 55, 64, 97, 139–40
    aftercare programme 27, 141
    cause of increased paperwork 277
direct patient care 79–84
    by nursing assistants 122–7
    defined 38
    effect of increased administration and
        paperwork 113–22
discharge and aftercare 27–8, 140–1
    assessment for 141, 142, 281
    blocked by lack of accommodation
        63, 281
    detained patients 141
    early discharge 27, 64, 140–1
    supervised discharge introduced 17
    uniformity of discharge process 140
    see also CPA
district general hospitals
    and age of patients 53
    and associated work 117, 118
    bed occupancy levels 48

bed provision 161
    and direct patient care 82, 84
    and paperwork 89
    and patient activities 136
    in pre-pilot study 35
    selected as fieldwork sites 32, 33
drug abuse 53–4, 54, 95, 157
dual diagnosis phenomenon 53

ECT treatment 72, 168–9
emotional cues 21, 26, 103–5
ethnic minority patients 54, 60, 61
    defined 49
evaluation 25, 107
    difficulty of measuring outcomes 278

feedback seminars 41–2
    reports 274–82
fieldwork *see* research methods
fieldwork sites 30–4
    hospital types selected 44, 45–6
    key characteristics 33, 45–56, 60–1
    problems in securing participation
        33–4
    statistical profiles 30–1
    see also Trust profiles
finance *see* cost, ward budgets

groupwork, therapeutic 107–8

HCAs *see* health-care assistants
health authorities
    issues for 155–6
health-care assistants (HCAs) 127, 131
'hierarchy of priority' 104
hospital managers, issues for 156–7
hospital types used in study *see under*
        fieldwork sites
    see also district general hospitals,
        inner-city hospitals

implementation of interventions 25
independent sector *see* private sector
indirect patient care 79–84
    by nursing assistants 122–7
    defined 38
inner-city hospitals
    and age of patients 53
    and associated work 116, 119

bed occupancy levels 48
and nurse-medical staff relations 87
and nurse-patient contact 84, 115, 138
and paperwork 89
and patient activities 136
patient populations 55, 60, 147
integrated patient notes 109, 153, 157

key worker (community) 141, 143
'key worker' in primary nursing 72

length of stay 17, 54
local authorities
mental health places 31, 169–71
recommendations for 155–6
relationship with hospitals 27–8, 276
see also community services

male-female patient ratio 52, 60, 61
MDT meetings 25, 108–10, 140, 152–3
medical staff
and MDTs 108–10
need to review roles 282
nurses' relationship with 87, 108,
153, 275, 278, 281
patients' attitudes to 139
shared role in admissions 96–7, 98
medication and changing role of nurse
20
MISG (Mental Illness Specific Grant) 16
mixed-sex wards 60
motivation of patients 102, 139
multidisciplinary working 22, 25,
108–10, 140, 141, 152–3, 157,
281–2
and accountability 277, 278
integrated patient notes 109, 153,
157
MDT meetings 25, 108–10, 140,
152–3

named nurse 23, 94, 99, 138–9, 277
and CPA 142, 143, 144, 145, 151
therapeutic relationship with patient
99–105, 112–13, 134–5
National Vocational Qualifications see
NVQs
nurse activity
questionnaire 36, 39, 245–52

schedule and glossary 215–17,
218–19, 222–3
nurse education see training
nurse expectations, need to clarify 148,
280
nurse interviews 36, 36–7, 186–207
nurse personal details questionnaire 36,
39, 248
nurse population 30–1, 34, 162–8
grades see D/E grade nurses, nursing
assistants, senior nurses
importance of grade mix 156
qualifications 128–30
shifts and working hours 67–72
nurse roles
administrative role see administration
and paperwork
in admission procedures 87, 96–7,
98, 99
counselling role 18–21, 19, 25,
110–12, 138–9, 275
in CPA 142, 143, 144, 145, 151, 152,
153
motivating role 102, 139
psychotherapeutic role 18–22
nurse skills
core skills 22
generic or specialist? 276
recommended separation of skills 155
see also training
nurse-patient relationship 25–6, 134–5
emotional cues 21, 26, 103–5
see also direct patient care, named
nurse
nursing assistants 26–7, 72
interview questions 193–6, 207–10
observation of patients 26
qualifications of those in the study
128–30
role and activities 98, 122–8, 153–4,
279
training 131
nursing staff numbers see nurse population
NVQs (National Vocational
Qualifications) 27, 127, 131, 158

observers/researchers 37–9
in pilot project 234, 235

occupational therapists 168, 282

paperwork *see* administration and paper-
    work
patient activities 135–8, 154
    schedule and glossary 215–21
patient expectations, need to clarify 148,
    157, 280–1
patient interviews 36, 210–14
patient mix 60, 147–8, 151, 277
patient perceptions
    of care plans 134
    of CPA 144–5
    of MDTs 109–10
    of named nurse's counselling role
        138–9
    of non-nursing staff 139
    of nurse-patient relationship 26,
        134–5
    of nursing care 133–5, 154
patient populations 47–55, 147–8
    difficult v. manageable 60–5
    obtaining data on 34–5
    regional differences 65
    see also patient mix
patient profile questionnaire 36, 39, 244
physiotherapists, numbers of (1988) 168
pilot project 35–6, 232–43
    see also pre-pilot studies
postal survey 40–1
    questionnaire 260–73
    see also Trust profiles
Powell, Enoch 14
pre-pilot studies 35, 224–31
primary nursing 72–4
private sector provision 31, 161–2
Project 2000 130–1, 276
Psychiatric Monitor System 133
Psychiatric Nursing: Today and Tomorrow
    (1968) 18–21, 22

qualifications, nursing 128–30
    see also NVQs

re-admission 53, 281
relapse management 149, 282
research and development of service 278
research methods 29–42
    analysis of data 39

feedback seminars 41–2, 274–82
fieldwork plan 36, 184–5
observers/researchers 37–9, 234, 235
    see also fieldwork sites, pilot project,
        postal survey, pre-pilot studies
researchers/observers 37–9
    in pilot project 234, 235
resource centres 23, 78
risk, acceptable 24, 96
risk assessment and management 96–7,
    142, 148, 151, 157, 281

schizophrenia and other psychoses 55,
    147
self-harm 107
senior nurses (G and F grades) 22, 279
    administration and paperwork 150,
        156
    administrative or clinical role? 23,
        78–9, 90–1
    and admissions 87, 96–7
    clinical supervision 77, 149–50, 156
    qualifications of those in the study
        128–30
    relationship with medical staff 87, 275
    responsibility, accountability, author-
        ity 85–8
    responsibility for staff cover 67–8
    and service development 74–5
    shifts worked 68–72
    teaching role 131
    time spent in direct patient care
        79–84
    see also ward managers
service development 74–5
severely ill patients
    increase in numbers 63
    indicators 54–5
sex ratio of patients 52, 60, 61
shifts and working hours 67–72
sickness, staff *see* staff sickness and stress
staff sickness and stress 75, 76–7, 149,
    153, 156, 280
stress *see* staff sickness and stress
suicide, risk of 13
supervision registers 16, 27, 142–3
supervision of staff 279–80
support for patients 103
support for staff 75, 157, 277

teamworking *see* multidisciplinary working
training 128–31
    in counselling and psychotherapeutic
      care 19–22
    dearth of post-registration courses
      131
    dominance of medical model 20–1,
      130
    issues to be addressed 157–8
    long enough? 282
    managerial qualifications 88
    mismatch between training and prac-
      tice 148–50, 158, 276, 282
    of nursing assistants 131
trust, establishing 26, 101–2
Trust profiles 34–5, 40, 173–6
    postal survey 253–9

unqualified nursing staff *see* nursing
    assistants

ward budgets 87
ward clerks 91, 157

ward environment 43–7, 55, 60, 134
    list 177–9
    questionnaire 34
ward managers 22, 90, 274
    do they need to be nurses? 78, 274
    interview questions 186–93, 196–207
    questionnaire 34, 180–3
ward profile and operational routines
    questionnaire 40, 260–73
ward round: replaced by MDT meeting
    108
wards: specialist or generic? 282
'Water Tower' hospitals 14, 32, 33
    and associated work 116–17
    and bed occupancy levels 48
    and bed provision 160, 161
    and direct patient care 82
    numbers of severely ill 55
    and paperwork 89
    and patient activities 136
    in pre-pilot study 35
*Working in Partnership: A Collaborative
    Approach to Care* (1994) 18, 21–2